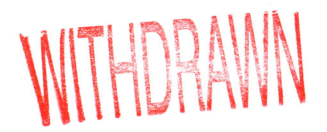

An Atlas of Investigation and Management

EPILEPSY

To my wife Priti and children Vikas and Tejas, who have been my inspiration and support, as well as all my friends, who have been the sunshine in my life.

D.N.

To my parents Michael and Patricia, whose love and support is never failing; and to my mentor Professor Soheyl Noachtar who, through his dedication, patience and enthusiasm, not only opened up the world of epilepsy for me, but also gave me a great love for it.

R.O'D.

An Atlas of Investigation and Management

EPILEPSY

Dileep R Nair, MD
Section Head of Adult Epilepsy
Director of Clinical Neurophysiology and
Intraoperative Neurophysiology Monitoring
Epilepsy Center
Neurological Institute
The Cleveland Clinic
Cleveland
USA

Rebecca O'Dwyer, MD
Epilepsy Research Fellow
Epilepsy Center, Neurological Institute
The Cleveland Clinic
Cleveland
USA

CLINICAL PUBLISHING
OXFORD

Clinical Publishing
an imprint of Atlas Medical Publishing Ltd
Oxford Centre for Innovation
Mill Street, Oxford OX2 0JX, UK

Tel: +44 1865 811116
Fax: +44 1865 251550
Email: info@clinicalpublishing.co.uk
Web: www.clinicalpublishing.co.uk

Distributed in USA and Canada by:
Clinical Publishing
30 Amberwood Parkway
Ashland OH 44805, USA

Tel: 800-247-6553 (toll free within US and Canada)
Fax: 419-281-6883
Email: order@bookmasters.com

Distributed in UK and Rest of World by:
Marston Book Services Ltd
PO Box 269
Abingdon
Oxon OX14 4YN, UK

Tel: +44 1235 465500
Fax: +44 1235 465555
Email: trade.orders@marston.co.uk

A catalogue record for this book is available from the British Library

ISBN-13   978 1 904392 54 5
ISBN e-book   978 1 84692 597 9

Project manager: Gavin Smith, GPS Publishing Solutions, Herts, UK
Illustrations by Graeme Chambers, BA(Hons)
Typeset by Phoenix Photosetting, Chatham, Kent, UK
Printed and bound by Marston Book Services Ltd, Abingdon, Oxon, UK

Contents

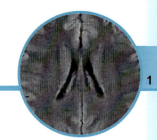

Chapter 1

An Introduction to Epilepsy

Introduction

Epilepsy is one of the most common neurological disorders. The need to accurately evaluate and treat seizures is within the realm of many physicians, including neurologists, internists, family doctors, paediatricians, geriatricians, emergency room physicians and obstetricians just to name a few. Seizures can present as a symptom in outpatient clinics as well as in hospitalized patients. Epilepsy affects a broad age group, has a diverse spectrum of aetiologies, and has a variable response to treatment. As one can imagine, making a diagnosis of epilepsy poses several challenges. The diagnosis is made with the highest degree of confidence when seizures are recorded during a video-electroencephalography (EEG) evaluation. For most patients who present with a history of seizures, results from video-EEG testing is usually not available and so the diagnosis is made using other available information. A careful and comprehensive history often enables an accurate diagnosis of epilepsy or may suggest the need for further testing, as well as helping to guide treatment decisions. The historical information comes from both the patient as well as from observers who have seen a patient's seizures. Whereas many additional tests such as neuroimaging and EEG may well be indicated in the evaluation of epilepsy, the importance of history cannot be overemphasized. Throughout this chapter and subsequent chapters in this atlas, various aspects of epilepsy will be highlighted. The intent of this atlas is for physicians to use it as a resource for a quick and easy guide for the assessment and diagnosis of various forms of epilepsy. There are some brief references in regards to the treatment of epilepsy, but this is not the main intent of this atlas.

Epidemiology

Every year 20 people in 100 000 will have had a seizure. For the majority, it will be their first and only seizure. A diagnosis of epilepsy can only be made when there has been at least two unprovoked seizures or recurring seizures with more than a 24-hour interval between each seizure. Epilepsy is a disease that knows no geographical, racial or social borders. The disorder affects the sexes equally with an approximate prevalence of 7.1 per 1000 people. The annual incidence has been reported to be 48 per 100 000 people with a higher incidence noted in developing countries, possibly due to poorer nutrition, hygiene and perinatal care, as well as an increased risk of cerebral infection.

The incidence of epilepsy peaks in infancy as well as in individuals over 60 years of age. Approximately 1% of the US population meets the diagnostic criteria for epilepsy but the actual prevalence may be significantly higher. Within 5 years of onset of seizures, 50–60% of patients will have entered a long period of remission. Up to 30% of patients will develop medically refractory epilepsy, despite multiple anticonvulsant medication trials. The standardized mortality rate associated with epilepsy is increased two to three times, with the excess mortality often directly linked to seizures. Compared with the general population, patients with epilepsy are more likely to be involved in accidents and suicides. Patients with epilepsy are also at greater risk of sudden unexpected death; it is estimated that there is one death per 250 people with severe and refractory epilepsy.

Useful definitions

- *Epileptic seizure*: a clinical manifestation that results from abnormal and excessive electrical discharges in a set of neurons within the brain. This may manifest as sudden or transitory alterations of consciousness, motor, sensory, autonomic or psychic events, which can be perceived by the patient or an observer.
- *Epilepsy*: a condition characterized by recurrent (two or more) epileptic seizures. Seizures occurring within a 24-hour period are considered as a single event.
- *Epileptic syndrome*: a further classification of the epilepsy that gives some information regarding the brain location from which the epilepsy arises. For example, if the epilepsy arises from the frontal lobes then the epilepsy syndrome is said to be frontal lobe epilepsy. If the epilepsy appears to have a generalized or widespread onset it may characterized as generalized epilepsy.
- *Seizure semiology*: the symptomatology occurring directly before, during and directly after a seizure.
- *Status epilepticus*: a single epileptic seizure of longer than 30 minutes or a cluster of epileptic seizures lasting for 30 minutes or longer during which the patient has not regained their baseline level of functioning.
- *Non-epileptic events*: episodic events that are not related to epileptic abnormal/excessive discharges. Aetiologies for non-epileptic events include (a) disturbances in the brain function (vertigo, dizziness, syncope, sleep and movement disorders, transient global amnesia, migraine and enuresis), and (b) pseudoseizures (non-epileptic sudden behavioural episodes presumed to be of psychogenic origin.
- *Ictal*: the period of time during an epileptic seizure.
- *Interictal*: the periods of time in between epileptic seizures.

Age frequency

The majority of people with newly diagnosed epilepsy are paediatric patients younger than age 2 or adults older than 65 years of age (**1.1**). Approximately 25% of new cases of epilepsy occur in women and men over the age of 60. There are no significant differences seen between the sexes.

Seizure types

The classification of epilepsies is a controversial subject. There are many classification systems including the

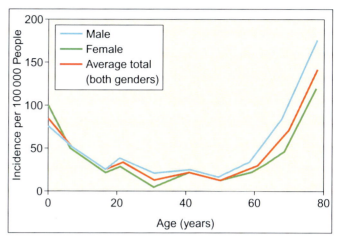

1.1 Incidence of epilepsy per 100 000 people.

International League Against Epilepsy (ILEA) classification (described further on pp. 11–13). Currently the classification is undergoing some revision. In obtaining an historical account of the seizure it is important to obtain the description from both the patients and observers. The patient's account will allow a description of various aura and symptoms prior to the loss of awareness or consciousness if they occur. The observer's description will give information during periods where the patient has no memory of the seizure. The descriptions are grouped under major headings based on various classification systems. The seizure classification described below includes terms being used currently in the ILAE classification as well as terms being used in the semiological classification (which has been advocated by some epilepsy centres around the world). The designation 'ILAE' for the ILAE classification or 'SE' for the semiological classification will denote terms specific to each classification system. One of the main disadvantages of the ILAE is that it is based not only on historical information but makes assumptions regarding the associated underlying epilepsy producing the seizure type, including on EEG data that may not be available (see below).

Aura

Auras occur at the beginning of a seizure and are only appreciated by the patient and are subjective symptoms. They usually are very brief and can occur in isolation. They are not detectable to the observer. Some examples of auras include: somatosensory auras (including tingling or alteration in sensation in a somatotopic distribution of the body); visual or auditory auras (can consist of hallucinations and illusions);

autonomic auras (can manifest with symptoms of tachycardia or goose bumps); abdominal auras (typically described as a rising sensation from the abdomen to the thorax or throat along with complaints of nausea); psychic auras (are complex and described as experiential symptoms of 'déjà vu', fear, or 'jamais vu'). The patient may exhibit some behavioural response during their aura, such as a fearful expression, which is simply a reaction to either the symptom of the aura or knowing that they are about to experience a seizure.

Dialeptic seizure (SE)

This term is used when there is an alteration of either consciousness or awareness as the major clinical manifestation of the seizure. Typically, the patient has no recollection of the seizure and their other associated motor manifestations. An absence seizure (ILAE) not only has an alteration of consciousness but also requires that whatever electroclinical information is available suggests that the seizure arose from generalized epilepsy.

Motor seizure (SE)

This terminology is used for seizures that have some significant motor component.

Simple motor seizures (SE) are those that comprise involuntary movements that bear no resemblance to physiological or natural movements. These movements can be elicited through stimulation of the primary motor cortex (Brodmann's area 4 and 6) or the supplementary sensorimotor area (Brodmann's area 6). At the beginning of these seizures consciousness may be preserved; however, it may be lost as the seizure develops.

In complex motor seizures (SE) they comprise complex movements that appear physiological, such as bicycling or moving about. However, these movements are inadequate or inappropriate for the patient's setting. During these seizures awareness is usually, although not always, altered.

Clonic seizures (SE and ILAE—although a prefix term 'generalized' is typically used in the ILAE classification)

These seizures consist of periodic, repetitive, short contractions of various muscle groups. Often these movements are found in the distal extremities, face or tongue. Epileptic discharges from the primary motor region (area 4) or the premotor region (area 6) lead to these movements. In the semiological classification clonic seizures may involve the entire body, when it is called generalized, or may be more limited, such as

involving only the left arm, in which case it would be termed left arm clonic seizure. This also holds true for tonic seizures.

Tonic seizure (SE and ILAE—although a prefix term 'generalized' is typically used in the ILAE classification)

These seizures comprise a persistent contraction of one or more muscle groups, which lead to tonic posturing. They most often appear in the proximal musculature and have a preference for the contralateral side to the epileptic focus. Epileptic stimulation of the supplementary sensorimotor region (medial area 6) leads to these movements.

Generalized tonic–clonic seizure (SE and ILAE)

This seizure type describes what has become known in the vernacular as 'grand-mal seizure'. It denotes a generalized seizure with semiology combining a generalized clonic seizure with a generalized tonic seizure.

Generalized atonic seizure (SE and ILAE)

This seizure type also denotes a seizure in which all motor tone is lost and the patient drops to the floor. Patients with these seizures are more prone to serious head injuries.

Myoclonic seizures (SE and ILAE—although a prefix term 'generalized' is typically used in the ILAE classification)

These seizures comprise of isolated, quick twitches, which can be generalized or focal in nature.

Versive seizures (SE)

These seizures consist of a forced unnatural turning of the heads and or eyes in one direction. The movement may be a smooth tonic contraction or be clonic. The deviation of the head and/or eyes may sometimes be followed by turning the trunk in the same direction. The important feature of this seizure type is that the movement leads to an unnatural, tonic posturing, which helps differentiate it from other non-versive head movements.

Complex partial seizure (ILAE)

A seizure in which consciousness is impaired, and electroclinical information suggests that the seizure arises from a focal epilepsy.

Hypomotor seizure or behavioural arrests

Patients during these seizures demonstrate reduced motor activity, although certain complex motor actions are still possible such as sitting upright or a blank stare. However, consciousness cannot be tested in this group of patients either because of mental disability or because of their young age.

Automotor seizures or complex partial seizures

Automatisms are involuntary, organized movements, such as miction, swallowing or nose rubbing. In the setting of these seizures the automatisms appear inappropriate to the patient's setting.

Hypermotor seizures or complex partial seizures

These seizures are characterized by a series of complex motor movements in the proximal extremities that appear fervid and sometimes even violent or bizarre. Automatisms are not observed in these seizures.

Risk factors

Complex febrile seizures

These seizures last more than 15 minutes with a predominantly unilateral symptomatology that recur within a single infection. They are usually associated with a rapid increase in temperature due to a viral illness. Approximately one-third of all febrile seizures are complex, usually occurring very early in the infection and may be the first clinical manifestation. They can, however, have a genetic basis and genetic studies have shown an autosomal dominant inheritance pattern of the SCN1A gene in families with generalized epilepsy and febrile seizures. Two to 10% of children with a history of febrile seizures will develop epilepsy later in life, in comparison with 0.5% of children with no history. It should be noted, however, that the risk for development of epilepsy is greater in children with a pre-existing neurodevelopmental dysfunction and the febrile seizure may be the first clue to their predisposition to epilepsy.

Head trauma

Injuries of this type can be divided into open and closed head trauma. Post-traumatic epilepsy occurs much more frequently with open head trauma, and the risk is greatest if damage occurs in large areas or involves frontal and temporal lobes, with 50–60% of patients experiencing their first (late) within the first 12 months after injury. Dural breach, encephalomalacia, intracranial haematoma and long post-traumatic amnesia have all been found to increase the risk of developing epilepsy.

Closed head trauma can also increase the risk for developing epilepsy; however, mild injury is not associated with any increased risk. One to 4% of patients with moderate injury, defined as head injury complicated by skull fracture or more than 30 minutes of post-traumatic amnesia, will develop epilepsy. As many as 10–15% of patients with severe head trauma—head injury with post-traumatic amnesia longer than 24 hours, cerebral contusion or intracranial haematoma—will develop epilepsy.

Family history

It is important to identify other family members who have been diagnosed with epilepsy because an increased prevalence has been established in affected families, which is consistent with both common environmental exposures as well as polygenic or multifactorial genetics. Cohort studies have shown there to be a two- to threefold increased risk of developing epilepsy in siblings and children of epileptics. The genetics of epilepsy will be discussed later.

Developmental delay

There has been an association between epilepsy and developmental delay, and careful history taking might hint towards an epileptic aetiology. In a paediatric study developmental delay or mental retardation was present in 37% of patients. Many of the aetiologies, such as cortical dysplasia, associated with paediatric epilepsy are also associated with cognitive impairment of varying degrees.

Some enzyme deficiency diseases may also lead to a developmental delay and be associated with epilepsy. These diseases often have a genetic basis and the exact mutation is known, which results in a protein dysfunction or deficiency, thus stunting cognitive development. Examples include Gaucher disease, Niemann–Pick disease type C, various lysosomal and peroxisomal disorders, porphyria, pyridoxone deficiency and Wilson disease.

Central nervous system infections

See *Table 1.1*.

Cerebrovascular disease

See *Table 1.2*.

Central nervous system tumours

See *Table 1.3*.

Seizure precipitants

See *Table 1.4*.

Table 1.1 The most common central nervous system infections and their most common infectious agent, which are associated with an increased risk for epilepsy. Chronic epilepsy is seven times more prevalent among people following meningitis or encephalitis than the general population

Disease	Common infective agents
Meningitis	*Streptococcus pneumoniae*
	Neisseria meningitides
	Haemophilus influenzae Type b
Encephalitis	Viral: herpes simplex type 1, 2 and 6;* cytomegalovirus;* Epstein–Barr virus; varicella;* measles,* mumps, rubella;* arboviruses; HIV; enterovirus; JC virus*
	Bacterial: (uncommon) *Borrelia burgdorferi*; *Brucella* spp.; *Mycobacterium tuberculosis*;* *Mycoplasma pneumoniae*;* *Rickettsia rickettsii*; *Treponema pallidum*; Protozoal*: (uncommon) Amoebic meningoencephalitis;* toxoplasmosis
	Fungal*: (uncommon) *Cryptococcus neoformans*;* coccidoidomycosis; blastomycosis; histoplasmosis; asperigillus; *Candida*
Cerebral malaria	*Plasmodium falciparum*
Pyogenic cerebral abscess	*Streptococci* spp.
	Bacteroides
	Gram-negative bacilli
	Clostridia spp.
	*Actinomyces**
	*Nocardia**
Neurocysticerosis	*Taenia solium*
Tuberculoma	*Mycobacterium tuberculosis**

*Infective agents more commonly found among immunocompromised patients.

Comorbidities

Epilepsy is associated with several comorbidities that impair patient health and the proper management of a patient with epilepsy includes treating these as well as gaining control over seizures. Approximately 5% of all annual visits to the emergency department are related to injuries as a result of seizures, such as head trauma, burns, falls and lacerations. Most other common comorbidities fall under three broad headings: psychiatric, cognitive impairment and endocrine dysfunction. There is a much higher rate among epileptics in comparison with the general population of anxiety disorders (19–66%) and depression (20–57%). These disorders probably have several aetiologies and are related to the disease pathology itself, the sedative effects of antiepileptic drugs (AEDs), as well as the psychosocial stigma appointed to seizures. Cognitive impairment has already been dealt with under 'Developmental delay'. Female patients with epilepsy are more likely to experience reproductive endocrine dysfunction than are female patients without epilepsy. Ovulatory dysfunction and hyperandrogenism in the absence of thyroid or adrenal disease usually takes the form of polycystic syndrome and is a common comorbidity among female patients. Other reproductive difficulties may arise from treatment with certain AEDs, which can reduce sexual drive and have teratogenic properties on the fetus. Epileptics are more likely to suffer from insulin resistance, diabetes mellitus type 2, hypertension, dyslipidaemia and cardiovascular disease; the exact pathophysiology has not been determined but probably involves neuroendocrine effects of seizures and/or AEDs.

Table 1.2 Brief overview of clinically important vascular malformations, which may be considered risk factors for epilepsy. Other diseases causing cerebrovascular lesions must not be forgotten, such as rheumatic heart disease, endocarditis, mitral valve prolapse or after post-carotid endarterectomy. There is also an association between arterial hypertension, eclampsia, hypertensive encephalopathy and malignant hypertension

Cerebrovascular disease	Increased risk for epilepsy
Haemorrhage	
Within first week	30%
Subarachnoid	20–34%
Overall	5–10%
Infarction	
Within 12 months	6%
Within 5 years	11%
Occult degenerative cerebrovascular disease	5–10%
Arteriovenous malformations	
Age: 10–19 years	44%
20–29 years	31%
30–60 years	6%
Cavernous haemangioma	40–70%
Venous malformations	NS
Vasculitides, e.g. systemic lupus erythematosus*	25%

NS, not significant.
*Epilepsy has also been associated with Behçet disease, Sjörgen syndrome, mixed-connective tissue disease and Henoch–Schönlein purpura among other vasculitides that affect the central nervous system.

Table 1.3 Brief overview of clinically important central nervous system (CNS) tumours, which are associated with epilepsy. Six per cent of all newly diagnosed cases of epilepsy are a result of a CNS neoplasm. This diagnosis is greatest in adults with approximately 25% of all new focal cases linked to a tumour. Seizures are seen in approximately 50% of all patients with brain tumour. Metastases from other primary tumours are also a source of epileptic foci and should also be considered

CNS tumour	Percentage of patients with epilepsy
Glioma	
Oligodendrogliomas	92%
Astrocytomas	70%
Glioblastomas	37%
Ganglioma	80–90%
Dysembryoplastic neuroepithelial tumour	Up to 100%
Hamartoma	
Hypothalamic hamartoma	Up to 100%
Meningioma	20–50%

> **Table 1.4 Common precipitants for epileptic seizures. It is important to review common precipitants for seizures while taking a history; some patients only have seizures under certain circumstances. These precipitants may also lead to non-epileptic seizures, such as syncopal seizures**

Common precipitants	Less common precipitants
Sleep deprivation and fatigue	Hormonal changes
Alcohol and alcohol withdrawal	Dietary changes
Photic stimulation	Fasting
Hyperventilation	Pain
Menstrual cycle	Allergies
Emotional disturbance	Startle
Stress	Sexual intercourse
Sleep–wake cycle	
Hypoglycaemia	
Metabolic disturbances	
Toxins and drugs	
Fever or ill health	

Differential diagnosis

The following is a list of the clinically most important differential diagnoses for epilepsy and should always be considered and ruled out:

- sleep disorders, e.g. narcolepsy, parasomnias
- transient ischaemic attack
- transient global amnesia
- migraine
- syncope
- vasovagal syndrome
- hypoglycaemia
- neoplasm with/without metastases
- neuroleptic malignant syndrome
- thyrotoxicosis
- attention deficit hyperactivity disorder
- conversion disorder
- narcotic overdose.

Physical examination

Usually the physical examination is benign, the important exception being when a structural cerebral lesion is involved. Therefore, care should be taken to detect any lateralizing signs, such as a positive Babinski sign, hyperreflexia or weakness, all of which may allude to an underlying structural lesion in the brain.

The physical examination may also help identify a possible aetiology. Often patients with neurocutaneous syndromes will appear in an epilepsy clinic and through the physical examination many of the required criteria for diagnosis may be easily identified.

Tuberous sclerosis
Tuberous sclerosis (TSC) is inherited in an autosomal fashion and usually caused by mutations in the TSC1 or TSC2 genes, both tumour suppressor genes (*Table 1.5, Table 1.6*). While this condition falls within the neurocutaneous syndromes, it is also a form of cortical dysplasia and the tubers appear histologically very similar to focal cortical dysplasia. Epilepsy is the presenting symptom in over 80% of all patients, either presenting in the neonatal period as West or Lennox–Gastaut syndromes, or later as adult onset partial or generalized epilepsy.

Neurofibromatosis type 1
Neurofibromatosis type 1 is inherited dominantly with practically complete penetrance, although half of the presented cases are due to spontaneous mutations. The incidence of epilepsy in these patients is 5–10%, taking various forms and presenting at any age.

Table 1.5 Necessary criteria to be fulfilled for diagnosis

Major features	Minor features
Facial angiofibromas or forehead plaque	Bone cysts
Non-traumatic ungula or periungual fibromas	Multiple pits in dental enamel
Hypomelanotic macules (3≥)	Hamartomas rectal polyps
Shagreen patch (connective tissue naevus)	Gingival fibromas
Multiple retinal nodular hamartomas	Cerebral white matter radial migration lines
Cortical tuber	Retinal achromic patch
Subependymal nodule	Non-renal hamartoma
Subependymal giant cell astrocytoma	'Confetti' skin lesions
Cardiac rhabdomyoma, single or multiple	Multiple renal cysts
Renal angiomyolipoma	
Lymphangiomyolipoma	

Definite TSC: Two major features or one major feature plus two minor features.
Probable TSC: One major feature plus one minor feature.
Possible TSC: One major feature or two or more minor features.

Table 1.6 Criteria required for diagnosis

Two or more of the following are required:

- ≥6 *café au lait* macules; diameter >5 mm in prepubertal individuals
- diameter >15 mm in postpubertal individuals
- ≥2 neurofibromas of any type or one plexiform neurofibroma
- Freckling in axillary or inguinal areas
- Optic glioma
- ≥2 Lisch nodules
- Bone lesions, e.g. thinning of long bone cortex, sphenoid dysplasia, pseudarthrosis
- First-degree relative diagnosed with neurofibromatosis 1

Sturge–Weber syndrome

The collection of symptoms that define the Sturge–Weber syndrome consist of unilateral or bilateral port-wine naevus, epilepsy, hemiparesis, mental impairment and ocular signs. Often epilepsy is the first symptom and at least 70% of patients develop epilepsy by their fourth birthday.

Many diseases associated with dysmorphisms are also associated with epilepsy and it is important to correctly identify these patients and the underlying pathology for effective treatment.

Epilepsy is present in up to 12% of all patients with Down syndrome. Other disorders of chromosome structure that are associated with epilepsy and dysmorphisms include fragile X syndrome and Ring chromosome 20.

Patients with anomalies in cortical development, often present with dysmorphisms and epilepsy. Apart from imaging, karyotyping and further genetic testing should be performed. Other such diseases include lissencephaly, anencephaly, agyria, agenesis of the corpus callosum and periventricular nodular heterotopia.

Aetiology

Many of the aforementioned risk factors may also be seen as aetiologies for epilepsy. With the advancement of modern molecular biology and neuroimaging, it is now becoming possible to identify new aetiologies of epilepsy.

Genetic

The genetics of epilepsy can be divided into four broad groups according to inheritance and phenotype (see *Tables 1.7–1.9*); the lists are by no means complete but try to report the most important advances in this field.

Abbreviations

AEDs   antiepileptic drugs
BECTS benign partial epilepsy with centro-temporal spikes
BFNC   benign familial neonatal convulsions
BMEI   benign myoclonic epilepsy of infancy
CAE   childhood absence epilepsy
CSWS   continuous spikes and waves during slow sleep
CT   computed tomography
EcoG   electrocorticography
EEG   electroencephalography
EGMA   epilepsy with *grand mal* on awakening
EMA   epilepsy with myoclonic absences
FDG   [^{18}F] fluoro-2-deoxy-D-glucose
FLAIR fluid attenuated inversion recovery
GTCS   generalized tonic–clonic seizure
IGE   idiopathic generalized epilepsy
ILEA   International League Against Epilepsy

JAE   juvenile absence epilepsy
JME   juvenile myoclonic epilepsy
LKS   Landau–Kleffner syndrome
MRI   magnetic resonance imaging
mTLE   mesial temporal lobe epilepsy
nTLE   neocortical temporal lobe epilepsy
PET   positron emission tomography
REM   rapid eye movement
SE   semiological classification
SPECT single photon emission computed tomography
SSC   seizure semiology classification
SSMA   supplementary sensorimotor area
SSME   supplementary sensorimotor epilepsy
SWC   spike–wave complexes
TLE   temporal lobe epilepsy
TSC   tuberous sclerosis

Acknowledgements

The authors would like to acknowledge the support and help of all members of the Epilepsy Center of the Cleveland Clinic, in particular the director of the center, Imad M. Najm, MD.

Preface

The main focus of this atlas is to give an overview of epilepsy to clinicians and trainees in the field of neurology and general medicine. The text covers various types of epilepsies including their clinical presentations, investigations, and management strategies. Numerous figures accompany the text to help give a more visual guidance in the learning process. In addition, there are extracts from EEG tracings that are meant to serve as examples of typical EEG features in the various forms of epilepsies that are discussed. Several clinical cases are also discussed to help guide the reader in gaining a better understanding of the various clinical and EEG manifestations of epilepsy.

This atlas is not meant to be an exhaustive review of epilepsy but rather serve as an introduction to the main 'themes' associated with the management of epilepsy. The book begins with introduction into the general issues that are important to the overall understanding of epilepsy such as epidemiology, frequently used terms, seizure types, risk factors, physical examination and aetiologies. Subsequent chapters are divided according to the various types of epilepsy based on localization – generalized, frontal, temporal. Each of these chapters has a similar format: an introduction is followed by a review of anatomy, seizure semiology, EEG features, neuroimaging and aetiologies. Each chapter then ends with case studies that help give a clinical meaning to the information provided. The last chapter discusses management strategies both in terms of broad concepts as well as relating to specific forms of epilepsy.

Dileep R Nair, MD
Rebecca O'Dwyer, MD
December 2009

Table 1.10 1981 International League Against Epilepsy (ILAE) Classification of Seizure Type

I Partial (focal, local) seizures
A Simple partial seizures
1 With motor signs
2 With somatosensory or special sensory symptoms
3 With autonomic symptoms or signs
4 With psychic symptoms
B Complex partial seizures
1 Simple partial onset followed by impairment of consciousness
2 With impairment of consciousness at onset
C Partial seizures evolving to secondarily generalized seizures (tonic–clonic, tonic or clonic)
1 Simple partial seizures evolving to generalized seizures
2 Complex partial seizures evolving to generalized seizures
3 Simple partial seizures evolving to complex partial seizures evolving to generalized seizures
II Generalized seizures (convulsive and non-convulsive)
A Absence seizures
1 Absence seizures
2 Atypical absence seizures
B Myoclonic seizures
C Clonic seizures
D Tonic seizures
E Tonic–clonic seizures
F Atonic seizures (astatic seizures)
III Unclassified epileptic seizures

Table 1.11 Seizure semiological classifications of epileptic seizures

Epileptic seizure
Aura
    Somatosensory aura*
    Auditory aura*
    Olfactory aura
    Abdominal aura
    Visual aura*
    Gustatory aura
    Autonomic aura*
    Psychic aura

Autonomic seizure*
Dialeptic seizure†
    Typical dialeptic seizure†
Motor seizure*
    Simple motor seizure*
        Myoclonic seizure*
        Epileptic spasm*
        Tonic–clonic seizure
        Tonic seizure*
        Clonic seizure*
        Versive seizure*
    Complex motor seizure†
        Hypermotor seizure†
        Automotor seizure†
        Gelastic seizure
Special seizure
    Atonic seizure*
    Hypomotor seizure†
    Negative myoclonic seizures*
    Astatic seizures
    Akinetic seizure*
    Aphasic seizure†
Paroxysmal event

*Left/right/axial/generalized/bilateral asymmetric.
†Left hemisphere/right hemisphere.

When taking a history it often proves difficult to report seizure symptoms with precision and accuracy. The SSC, by following a hierarchical progression, optimizes known semiological information and allows seizure classification of different degrees of precision. For example, if the patient had an epileptic seizure, it is classified as 'epileptic seizure'. If the seizure is characterized by motor manifestations, it is classified as 'motor seizure'. If the movements were 'simple' and predominantly in the right arm, however, no further description can be assigned to them; the seizure is then classified as 'right arm simple motor seizure'. However, if the movements are of a clonic type, the seizure is then classified as 'right arm clonic seizure'.

Further diagnostic studies

Laboratory screening
It is important to consider the patient's clinical picture and possible differential diagnoses, when deciding which values to

evaluate. A basic screen should include complete blood count, glucose, calcium, magnesium, thyroid-stimulating hormone, haematology studies, renal function tests and toxicology screen. If taken directly after a seizure, a metabolic acidosis and leucocytosis might be detected. Prolactin levels may rise shortly after a generalized tonic-clonic seizure and some partial seizures; however, even when compared with a baseline value taken 6 hours later, a prolactin level will not be able to distinguish an epileptic seizure from syncope.

Lumbar puncture

If the clinical picture is suggestive of an infectious aetiology or the patient has a history of cancer known to metastasize to the meninges, then after exclusion of increased intracranial pressure, a lumbar puncture should be performed and the appropriate cytology done.

Electroencephalography

EEG studies are an essential part of the epilepsy evaluation. A negative EEG study does not necessarily rule out epilepsy and many EEG findings are non-specific. Patients with migraines, encephalopathies and taking certain medications may also display abnormal EEG patterns. Usually, patients are asked to come to elective EEG studies sleep deprived, and may be subjected to periodic photic stimulation or asked to hyperventilate in order to provoke seizures.

Neuroimaging

For the identification of epileptic lesions, MRI is preferred over computed tomography (CT). A CT scan, however, is useful to exclude a mass lesion or haemorrhage. MRI scans should include proton density weighted, T1-weighted and T2-weighted images in axial, coronal and saggital planes (5 mm slices) (1.0 Telsa). If the MRI is normal, additional testing with high-resolution (1–3 mm slices) MRI with inversion recovery, 3D-fast low angle shot images, FLAIR 9and magnetization prepared rapid attenuated gradient echo could be performed (1.5 Telsa). Further imaging studies can be undertaken in selected patients, including interictal [18F] fluoro-2-deoxy-D-glucose positron emission tomography and ictal 99mTc-ethyl-cysteinate-dimer single photon emission CT following established protocols.

Treatment

The primary goals of treatment for epilepsy should include control of seizures—ideally achieving freedom from seizures—as well as minimizing the occurrence of adverse events, including those arising from drug–drug interactions, and improving the patient's quality of life. Comorbidities and psychosocial challenges can also affect the clinical course of epilepsy and need to be considered in tailoring treatment strategies to the needs of the individual patient.

Medical treatment

Pharmacotherapy is a key component of epilepsy management. Over the last 10 years, a variety of AEDs have been introduced, making it possible to tailor treatments to an individual patient's needs.

1.4 depicts the place of action of the newer AEDs at the synapse. They tend to work at voltage-gated ion channels, where they can enhance inhibitory neurotransmitters or reduce excitatory neurotransmission.

Antiepileptic drug indications
See *Table 1.12*.

Treatment strategies
Experts agree that monotherapy as the first-line treatment for epilepsy is to be recommended. In the event of failure of the first monotherapy, an alternative monotherapy is recommended as the second-line treatment. Should a second-line monotherapy fail, the experts are divided between the strategy of trying a third monotherapy and initiation of polytherapy with two AEDs (**1.5**).

If a second drug is added, the dose of the first drug may need to be adjusted because of drug–drug interactions. Should the patient become seizure free on polytherapy, the dose of the initial drug may be reduced in order to reduce the risk of side effects.

In tailoring antiepileptic treatment to the individual patient, factors such as seizure and epilepsy type, side effect profile, patient profile, ease of use of the antiepileptic medication and cost should be considered, with the aim of achieving the best balance among efficacy, tolerability and safety. Epilepsy is a chronic disease and patients may take antiepileptic medication for many years. Therefore, long-term as well as short-term efficacy and tolerability should be considered.

Side effects
Ideally, a seizure medication should prevent seizures without causing any side effects. The clinician should treat the patient with epilepsy with the appropriate medication

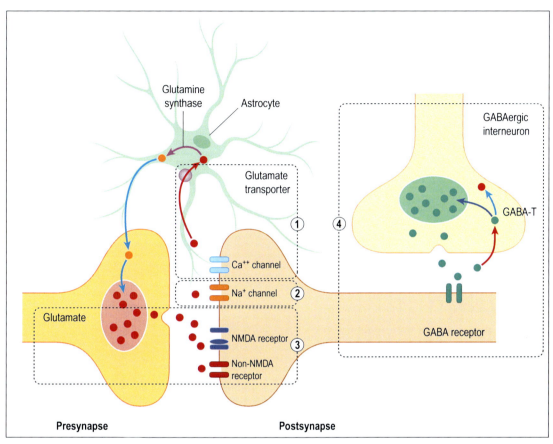

1.4 A schematic representation of the mode of action of common new antiepileptic drugs. 1. Calcium channel blockade: Felbamate, Lamotrigine, Topiramate, Zonisamide. 2. Sodium channel blockade: Felbamate, Lamotrigine, Oxcarbazepine, Topiramate, Zonisamide. 3. Antagonism of glutamate: Felbamate, Topiramate. 4. Potentiation of GABA activity: Tiagabine, Topiramate.

or combination of medications that provides optimum control of seizures with an acceptable level of side effects. Some of the prominent safety and tolerability issues to be considered in selecting an AED include: the potential for idiosyncratic reactions such as serious rash, hepatic toxicity and anaemia; neurological toxicity as manifested by symptoms such as drowsiness, dizziness, ataxia and tremor; long-term safety and tolerability as reflected in the potential for causing neuropathy, cosmetic effects and effects on bone; teratogenicity; and reproductive endocrine effects.

Surgical treatment

Before we discuss the concepts of epileptic surgery, first let us define some important regions in the epileptic brain, which will prove vital to understanding the concepts behind surgical treatment (**1.6**).

Subdivisions of epileptogenicity

The symptomatogenic zone is defined as the area of cortex, which, when activated by an epileptiform discharge, produces ictal symptoms. For this area of cortex to produce symptoms, the stimulus must have the appropriate frequency and be of sufficient duration and intensity. If the stimulus does not fulfil all these criteria, this zone will not elicit a response.

The epileptogenic zone is the area of cortex that is indispensable for the generation of epileptic seizures. The seizure onset zone is the area of cortex that actually generates clinical seizures. If the epileptogenic zone is smaller than the seizure onset zone, partial resection of the seizure onset zone may render the patient seizure free, as the remaining seizure onset zone is incapable of generating a seizure. However, if the epileptogenic zone is larger than the seizure onset zone, total resection of the seizure onset zone will not lead to

Table 1.12 The most common antiepileptic drugs (AEDs) and their indication

Indication/AED:	CBZ	KLN	ETX	GBP	LTG	LVT	OXC	PHB	PHT	PGB	PRM	TGB	TPM	VPA	VGB	ZNM
Partial seizures																
simple	yes	yes	no	yes	yes	yes	yes	yes	yes	yes	yes	(yes)	yes	yes	yes	yes
complex	yes	yes	no	yes	yes	yes	yes	yes	yes	yes	yes	(yes)	yes	yes	yes	yes
evolve to 2° GTC	yes	yes	no	yes	yes	yes	yes	yes	yes	yes	yes	(yes)	yes	yes	yes	yes
Generalized seizures																
absence	no	no	yes	no	yes	no	no	no	no	no	no	no	no	yes	no	no
myoclonic	no	yes	no	(yes)	no	(yes)	no	yes	no	no	yes	no	no	yes	no	(yes)
tonic–clonic	yes	(yes)	no	yes	yes	no	yes	yes	yes	no	yes	no	yes	yes	yes	yes
atonic	(yes)	(yes)	no	(yes)	(yes)	no	(yes)	(yes)	(yes)	no	(yes)	no	(yes)	yes	(yes)	(yes)

CBZ, Carbamazepine; ETX, Ethosuximide; GBP, Gabapentin; KLN, Clonazepam; LTG, Lamotrigine; LVT, Levetiracetam; OXC, Oxcarbazepine; PGB, Pregabalin; PHB, Phenobarbital; PHT, Phenytoin; PRM, Primidone; TGB, Tiagabine; TPM, Topiramate; VGB, Vigabatrin; VPA, Valproate; ZNM, Zonisamide. (yes) denotes that the drug may be used under restricted circumstances; however, further reading of the literature is required.

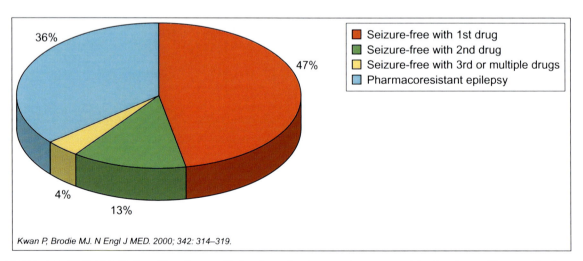

- Seizure-free with 1st drug
- Seizure-free with 2nd drug
- Seizure-free with 3rd or multiple drugs
- Pharmacoresistant epilepsy

Kwan P, Brodie MJ. N Engl J MED. 2000; 342: 314–319.

1.5 Approximately one-third of patients with epilepsy will develop refractory or pharmacoresistant epilepsy. These patients pose a particular challenge to physicians and usually further diagnostic tools and more invasive treatment strategies are required. None the less almost half of untreated patients will go into remission with their first antiepileptic drug.

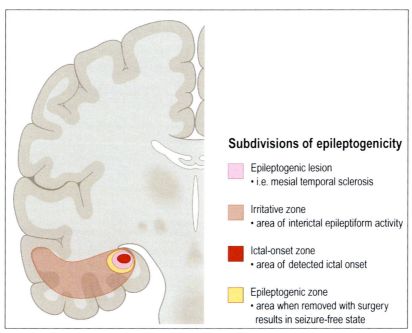

Subdivisions of epileptogenicity

Epileptogenic lesion
• i.e. mesial temporal sclerosis

Irritative zone
• area of interictal epileptiform activity

Ictal-onset zone
• area of detected ictal onset

Epileptogenic zone
• area when removed with surgery
  results in seizure-free state

1.6 A schematical representation of the different subdivisions of epileptogenicity.

seizure freedom. A seizure onset zone of a higher threshold within the epileptogenic zone may replace the resected zone and become clinically evident.

It is important to note that there is frequently no overlap between the symptomatogenic and epileptogenic zones. With the aid of EEG and neuroimaging, it is known that the epileptogenic discharge is generated in the epileptogenic zone and then spreads to the syptomatogenic zone, usually some distance from the epileptogenic zone.

The irritative zone is the region of cortex that generates interictal epileptiform discharges on EEG or magnetic encephalography.

The ictal onset zone is the region of cortex where clinical seizures are recorded to originate.

The ictal symptomatogenic zone is the region of cortex that generates the initial seizure symptomatology.

The region of cortex that remains abnormal during the inter-ictal period is known as the functional deficit zone. Neurological examination, neuropsychological testing, functional imaging or non-epileptiform EEG abnormalities may be used to identify the functional deficit zone.

Concepts of surgery

The aim of resective surgery is to remove the epileptogenic zone with preservation of eloquent cortex and thereby rendering the patient seizure free. Resective epilepsy surgery has proved to be a highly successful approach to treating patients with refractory epilepsy, rendering up to 70% seizure free in some situations. However, it should be noted that these patients have to be appropriately selected to ensure good surgical outcome (**1.7**).

It is important to assess these risks pre-operatively, in which neuropsychological testing plays a vital part. The Wada test is sometimes used to assess language and memory function in each hemisphere independently. The most common complication after a temporal lobectomy is impaired cognitive function. Generally there is a decrement in verbal IQ after left temporal lobe resection, although small increases in verbal and performance IQ has been noted after right temporal lobe resections. Other important complications are visual field deficits, usually found in the superior quadrant, after temporal lobectomy. In approximately 6% other neurological deficits may be seen, such as aphasia, cranial nerve palsy and hemiparesis, although they are permanent in only 50% of patients.

Vagus nerve stimulator

Patients who have refractory epilepsy and are not candidates for surgery may benefit from a vagus nerve stimulator (**1.9**). It was developed on the basis that intermittent stimulation of the vagus nerve can suppress seizures in experimental animals.

The stimulator is approximately 5 cm in diameter, it is surgically implanted subcutaneously on the lateral chest wall and connected to stimulating electrodes attached to the left vagus nerve in the neck by a wire tunnelled under the skin.

The stimulator certainly exerts some antiepileptic effect; however, as to how effective it is, remains debatable. This is probably due to the large number of possible variations in stimulation parameters, which make it difficult to study its effects systematically. It has been suggested that the antiepileptic effects may only be seen a few months after the initiation of treatment. It should also be considered that

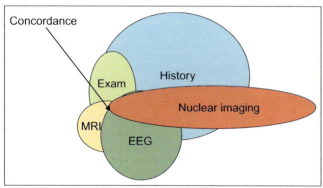

1.7 Concordant findings among the various diagnostic tools are vital to successful resective surgery. Successful resective surgery requires an accurate localization of the epileptogenic zone, a theoretical zone that despite modern technology cannot be measured directly. Therefore, it is necessary to utilize as many diagnostic tools as possible and infer from their concordant findings the localization of the epileptogenic zone (1.8). Resective surgery in patients with discordant findings will probably lead to persistent seizures following surgery.

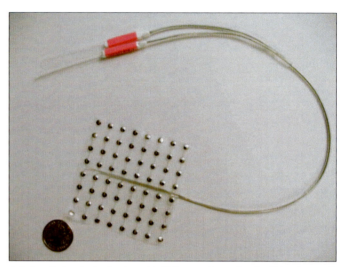

1.8 A subdural electrode grid. This consists of a flexible sheet of Silastic or Teflon with small electrodes (diameter 2–4 mm) made out of stainless steel, platinum, nichrome or silver embedded in it spaced 10 mm apart. These grids come in various sizes and shapes and can be cut to fit varying areas of cortex. Despite being only 1.5 mm thick, a craniotomy is required for placement.

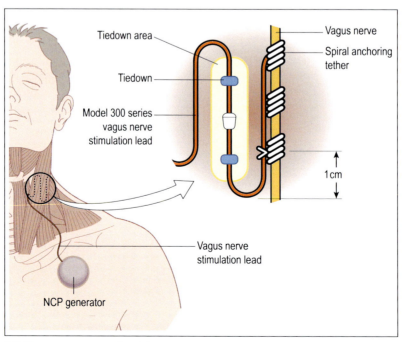

1.9 The vagus nerve stimulator.

after stimulator placement, the patient is prohibited from any CT, MRI or any other electromagnetic imaging studies, which might prevent them from possibly advantageous imaging studies in the future.

Further reading

Chang B, Lowenstein D. Mechanisms of disease epilepsy. *N Engl J Med* 2003; **349**; 1257–66.

Engle J Jr, Pedley TA (eds). *Epilepsy: A Comprehensive Textbook*. Associate ed., Aicardi J. Philadelphia: Lippincott-Raven; 1999.

Hauser WA, Annegers JF, Kurland LT. Incidence of epilepsy and unprovoked seizures in Rochester, Minnesota: 1935–1984. *Epilepsia* 1993; **34**(3): 453–68.

Kotagal P, Lüders HO (eds). *The Epilepsies: Etiologies and Prevention*. San Diego: Academic Press; 1999.

Lüders HO, Comair Y (eds). *Epilepsy Surgery*. New York: Lippincott, Williams and Wilkins; 2001.

Lüders HO, Noachtar S (eds). *Epileptic Seizures: Pathophysiology and Clinical Semiology*. New York: Saunders; 2000.

Shorvon SD (ed.). *Handbook of Epilepsy Treatment: Forms, Causes and Therapy in Children and Adults*, 2nd edn. Oxford: Wiley-Blackwell; 2005.

Chapter 2

The Generalized Epilepsies

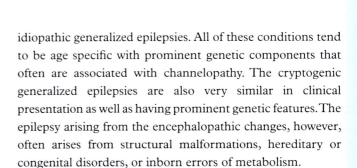

Introduction

Epileptic syndromes with seizures arising simultaneously from both hemispheres have been broadly named generalized epilepsy. This group may be further divided into two others based on their presumed aetiology: idiopathic generalized epilepsies and cryptogenic or symptomatic generalized epilepsies. They have a respective annual incidence of 6.65 and 1.15 per 100 000, accounting for 40% of all epilepsies and making up a higher proportion of all paediatric epilepsies. There is often a great overlap in symptoms between the various syndromes, although the aetiologies vary over a broad spectrum. *Table 2.1* lists the common clinical features of

idiopathic generalized epilepsies. All of these conditions tend to be age specific with prominent genetic components that often are associated with channelopathy. The cryptogenic generalized epilepsies are also very similar in clinical presentation as well as having prominent genetic features. The epilepsy arising from the encephalopathic changes, however, often arises from structural malformations, hereditary or congenital disorders, or inborn errors of metabolism.

Idiopathic generalized epilepsy (IGE) is a confusing term, referring to the fact there is no apparent structural cause and not meaning 'of unknown cause'. IGE probably has a genetic basis of polygenic origin with variable penetrance. IGE accounts for 10–20% of all cases of epilepsy and can be subdivided as shown in *Table 2.2*.

Juvenile myoclonic epilepsy (JME) is the most common subtype of IGE, accounting for 10% of all (both adult and paediatric) epilepsies. Its incidence peaks between the ages of 12 and 18 years; however, it is often not recognized by the patient or family initially and is mistaken for morning clumsiness, as seizures usually occur upon awakening or

Table 2.1 Shared clinical features of idiopathic generalized epilepsies

Onset in childhood/early adulthood	Family history
Normal electroencephalography background	Generalized seizure types
Diurnal pattern of seizure occurrence	Seizures exacerbated by hyperventilation or photosensitivity
Generalized electroencephalography discharges; spike and wave or polyspike bursts	Normal intellect and low comorbidity
Excellent prognosis under treatment with valproate	No identifiable underlying focal aetiology

Table 2.2 Subdivisions of idiopathic generalized epilepsies

- Juvenile myoclonic epilepsy
- Childhood absence epilepsy (pyknolepsy)
- Juvenile absence epilepsy
- Epilepsy with myoclonic absences
- Epilepsy with *grand mal* on awakening
- Benign familial neonatal convulsions
- Benign myoclonic epilepsy of infancy
- Myoclonic–astatic epilepsy
- Absence with peri-oral myoclonia

of each other. Both syndromes have a male preponderance and occur during cortical synaptogenesis; however, they have different peak ages of onset, with LKS at 2–7 years and CSWS at 3–5 years. LKS is characterized by developmentally normal children who present with a progressive aphasia, developing over months or subacutely over weeks. Some have argued that it is not an aphasia but an auditory agnosia; however, the children's verbal comprehension and expressive speech still remain severely affected. Children with CSWS present with similar symptoms; however, in 30% of cases a neurological pathology is already present and identified. Even after remission of seizures, most patients of both syndromes never return to their developmental or intellectual baseline, those with an earlier onset of spike–wave complexes (SWC) being the worst affected.

Seizure semiology

In generalized epilepsy syndromes, the seizure semiology may take many forms. It can either be non-convulsive, such as in absence and astatic seizures, or show convulsive motor semiology as in myoclonic, clonic, tonic and tonic–clonic seizures. It should be noted that there are no lateralizing signs, and movement occurs bilaterally and often symmetrically. Often similar seizure semiology is seen in many different subdivisions making it difficult to accurately define the syndrome.

Idiopathic generalized epilepsies

JME is initially characterized by myoclonic jerks occurring within approximately the first hour of waking and occurring in bursts. Eighty per cent of patients, months or years after the initial onset the myoclonus, may develop into GTCS, although these seizures usually occur infrequently (approximately twice in 1 year). Brief absence seizures, lasting approximately 15 s, are also seen in a third of patients.

In CAE the patient loses consciousness for approximately 10–15 s and is unresponsive or barely responsive to external stimuli. The patient has no recollection of the episode and because these seizures are so short they are often not recognized as seizures for long periods. They can occur many times during the day and tend to come in clusters. If the eyes are closed at onset, they open after 2–3 s. Automatisms are not uncommon, although they are not stereotyped and some retropulsive movements of the head and eyes may occur. The seizure semiology of JAE is similar in many

aspects to CAE; however, the impairment of consciousness is not as severe and the patient may maintain some mild awareness and responsiveness. Myoclonic jerks also occur, as well as occasionally GTCS, especially in seizures occurring after awakening or in provocative situations, such as sleep deprivation, after alcohol consumption or fatigue. The duration of the absences is also longer, lasting up to 21 s. As the name suggests, seizures in EMA are dominated by myoclonic absences, other seizures many infrequently include GTCS or falling attacks. An important difference in semiology compared with the other absence syndromes is that awareness of jerks may be maintained.

In EGMA the seizure type consists of GTCS without an aura during the first hour of awakening or evening period of relaxation. In some patients the GTCS is preceded by a series of absence or myoclonic seizures. Owing to the proximity with sleep, often the patient is amnestic of the seizure and the physician must rely on a history from a close relative.

In BFNC, seizures are characterized as focal or multifocal, clonic or tonic, and occurring during sleep. They are usually short, lasting from 1 to 3 min, and may recur until 2–3 months of age. As the name suggests, BMEI is characterized by massive generalized myoclonic seizures only, with a tendency for seizures to occur upon waking or when the child is falling asleep. Seizures can be prolonged especially if occurring during sleep or on waking, lasting up to 20 minutes in some cases.

Cryptogenic or symptomatic generalized epilepsies

The seizures of West syndrome include distinct infantile spasms, which take the form of sudden, general bilateral and symmetrical contractions of the muscles of the neck, trunk or limbs. As the condition evolves the spasms grow in frequency, peaking at several hundred per day. They also tend to come in clusters, with the intensity of spasm increasing and then dissipating within a cluster. The flexor muscles are predominantly affected, comprising of sudden flexion with both upper and lower limbs held in adduction (the so-called salaam attacks). Extensor spasms are less common; however, flexor–extensor spasms occur more commonly.

The Lennox–Gestaut syndrome displays a broad range of seizure types, including atypical absence, myoclonic, clonic, tonic and tonic–clonic seizures; these may then later develop into other seizure types, such as complex partial seizures. The most characteristic seizure type is the tonic seizure, occurring most often in non-REM (rapid eye movement) sleep and in wakefulness. These seizures usually lead to unprotected falls, referred to as 'drop attacks', and patients can sustain serious head, facial or orthopaedic injuries as a result. The other common seizure types are the atypical absence and tonic–clonic. Episodes of non-convulsive status epilepticus are also very common and may last from hours to days. During these periods consciousness may not be affected very much, although the patients might experience alterations in muscle tone, periodic myoclonic jerks or increased sialorrhoea.

Seizures in LKS vary greatly and most commonly consist of eye blinking with a brief eye deviation, head drop and minor automatisms followed occasionally by secondary generalization. Seizures in CSWS can occur in sleep, consisting of GTCS or myoclonic seizures and in wakefulness, consisting of either unilateral partial and then GTCS, absence seizures or atonic seizures.

Electroencephalography in generalized epilepsies

The EEG findings of seizure activity in generalized epilepsies can be divided into two broad patterns. The first pattern is characterized by a monomorphic, rhythmical, hypersynchronous 3 Hz SWC occurring in discrete bursts beginning at ictal onset (see **2.2**). Interictally the EEG is normal. This pattern is associated predominantly with absence seizures and represents alternating excitation and inhibition of the cortex. In absence seizures the inhibitory influences predominate and the negative clinical symptoms reflect this.

The second pattern is mainly associated with tonic–clonic seizures, starting with faster rhythmical frequencies that evolve to higher amplitude and slower frequencies. As ictal termination approaches, intermittent slow waves appear and become more frequent and prominent. The initial faster frequencies correlate to an excitatory phase of ictal generation and propagation, which later through increasing inhibitory influences result in ictal termination, the latter correlating to the increasingly prominent slow waves (**2.3**A–E). Generalized epileptiform discharges such as spikes, sharp waves and SWC are usually maximal bifrontally with typical phase reversals at F3 and F4.

Idiopathic generalized epilepsies

In JME, 50% of patients display abnormalities such as 3 Hz SWC or a faster polyspike–wave at 4–6 Hz associated with myoclonus. The EEG of approximately one-third of patients displays a photo-paroxysmal response. The background EEG

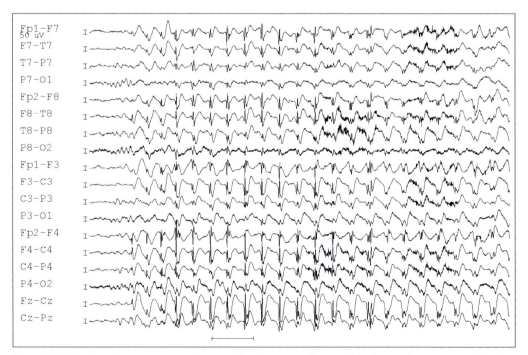

2.2 Displays the characteristic 3 Hz spike–wave complex seen in absence epilepsy. Note its regular monomorphic form and generalized distribution.

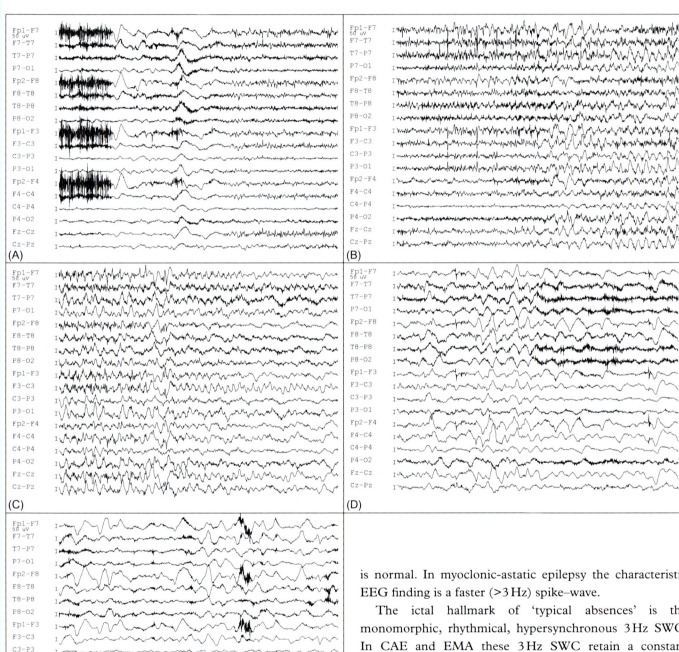

2.3 (A–E) The electroencephalography evolution in 10 s epochs (pages) of a generalized tonic–clonic seizure as described in the text.

is normal. In myoclonic-astatic epilepsy the characteristic EEG finding is a faster (>3 Hz) spike–wave.

The ictal hallmark of 'typical absences' is the monomorphic, rhythmical, hypersynchronous 3 Hz SWC. In CAE and EMA these 3 Hz SWC retain a constant relationship with slow waves, as well as the presence of generalized spikes or double spikes. The interictal EEG is normal or shows rhythmic posterior delta activity. Similar EEG characteristics are seen in JAE; however, polyspikes and discharge fragmentation are more common (**2.4**, **2.5**).

The most common EEG finding in EGMA is an increase in slow waves, disorganized background activity with sleep transients and generalized spike–wave activity. In sleep there is only a moderate increase in spike–wave activity.

The ictal EEG findings in BFNC are not particularly distinctive from other generalized seizure types. The interictal

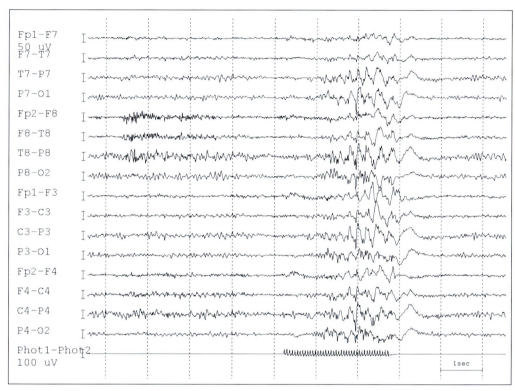

2.4 An example of generalized polyspikes induced by photostimulation in juvenile myoclonic epilepsy. In some patients, photostimulation may induce myoclonic seizures.

EEG pattern can be normal or display a rhythmic slow activity with discontinuous, multifocal sharp waves and hemispheric asynchrony. The seizure patterns of BMEI are characterized by brief generalized SWC and polyspikes, which are seen constantly when the child is falling asleep and in the first stages of sleep. Photostimulation can provoke seizure pattern changes and myoclonic seizures. The interictal EEG rarely shows any abnormalities during wakefulness; however, during sleep it shows generalized SWCs.

Cryptogenic or symptomatic generalized epilepsies

One of the defining characteristics of West syndrome is hypsarrhythmia (**2.6**) found on EEG. There is a continuous high-amplitude generalized slowing (during wakefulness) without any organized background and it is accompanied by multifocal spikes.

In the Lennox–Gastaut syndrome the ictal EEG findings vary depending on the type of seizure (**2.7**). There tend to be many similarities with the second pattern described above. A more irregular, slower SWC (<2.5 Hz) is seen than in absence epilepsy. These SWC also come in bursts;

however, they are less discrete and between them, other EEG abnormalities are seen. In atypical absence seizures it is sometimes difficult to distinguish from ictal and interictal EEG patterns. The background activity is abnormal with an excess of slow activity and decreased arousal or sleep potentials. During non-REM sleep, bursts of high frequency activity (>10 Hz) may be seen with or without a clinical tonic seizure.

Both LKS and CSWS display a distinctive 1.5–5 Hz spike–wave discharges in EEG in slow sleep that disappear or fragment in REM sleep. However, these spike–wave discharges are more prominent in the posterior temporal regions in LKS and in CSWS appear bilaterally in either a more focal or generalized manner (**2.8**).

Neuroimaging

Often, neuroimaging fails to find any underlying structural lesion in IGE. In cryptogenic generalized epilepsy, with improvements and advances in neuroimaging techniques the number of cryptogenic cases is dramatically decreasing.

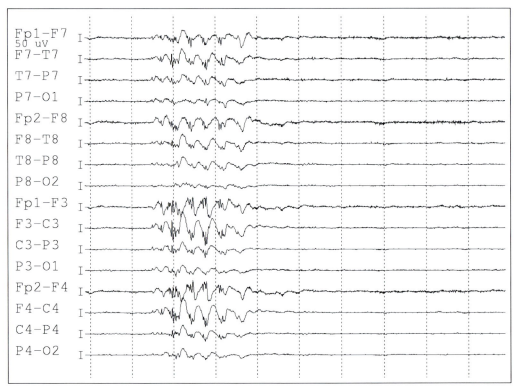

2.5 Another example of generalized polyspikes in juvenile myoclonic epilepsy; however, this time they were not induced by stimulation.

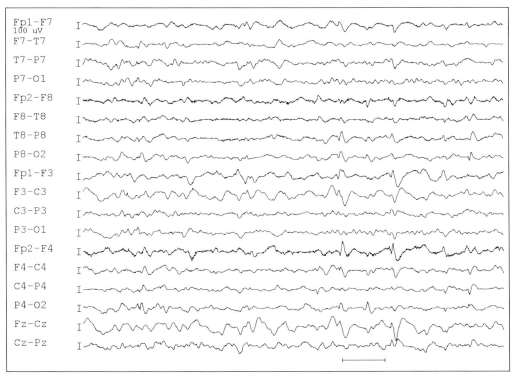

2.6 Demonstrates the characteristic hypsarrhythmia of West syndrome. An organized background cannot be identified; there is a constant, generalized slowing of high amplitude, accompanied by multifocal sharp waves.

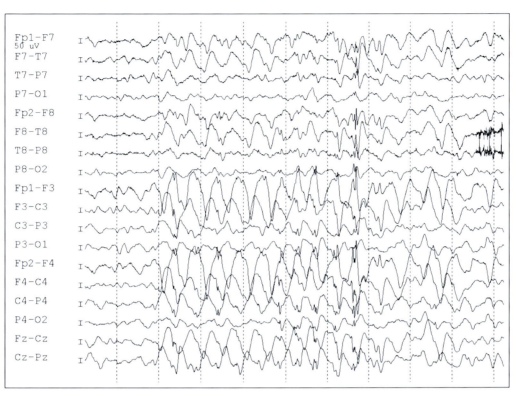

2.7 Generalized slow spike–wave complex with a frequency of approximately 2.5 Hz, as often seen in the Lennox–Gastaut syndrome.

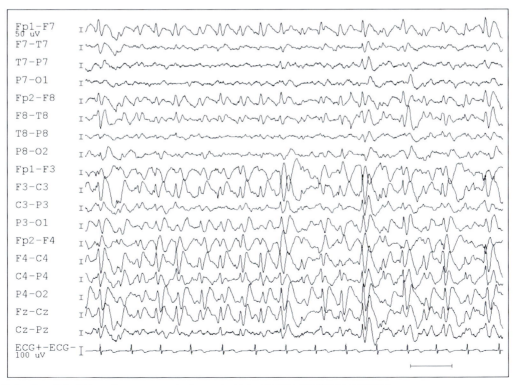

2.8 Displays the distinctive 1.5–5 Hz spike–wave complexes seen in Lindau–Kleffner syndrome.

Recent advances in high-resolution T1-weighted images and fluid-attenuated inversion recovery imaging has greatly helped to identify certain structural lesions in magnetic resonance imaging, such as cortical dysplasias. In West syndrome, for example, despite normal magnetic resonance imaging scans or ones diagnosed to have subtle dysplastic lesions, a positron emission tomography scan may help identify unifocal or multifocal lesions. Neuroimaging in LKS tends to be normal in comparison with CSWS, which usually displays evidence of a previous neurological insult. Possible structural abnormalities seen in LKS include focal pachgyria and mild diffuse atrophy. The aforementioned abnormalities as well as focal porencephaly and minor white matter abnormalities are seen in CSWS.

Conclusions

An overview of the important generalized epilepsies with all pertinent clinical information can be seen in *Table 2.4*.

Further reading

Engle J Jr, Pedley TA (eds). *Epilepsy: A Comprehensive Textbook*. Associate Ed., Aicardi J. Philadelphia: Lippincott-Raven; 1999.

Ferraro TN, Dlugos DJ, Buono RJ. Role of genetics in the diagnosis and treatment of epilepsy. *Expert Rev Neurother* 2006; **6**(12): 1789–800.

Gamble CL, Williamson PR, Marson AG. Lamotrigine versus carbamazepine monotherapy for epilepsy. *Cochrane Database Syst Rev*. 2006; Jan 25(1).

Lüders HO, Noachtar S (eds). *Epileptic Seizures: Pathophysiology and Clinical Semiology*. New York: Saunders; 2000.

Mohanraj R, Brodie MJ. Outcomes of newly diagnosed idiopathic generalized epilepsy syndromes in a non-pediatric setting. *Acta Neurol Scand* 2007; **115**(3): 204–8.

Nordli DR Jr, Korff CM, Goldstein J, Koh S, Laux L, Kelley KR. Cryptogenic late-onset epileptic spasms or late infantile epileptogenic encephalopathy? *Epilepsia* 2007; **48**(1): 206–8.

Shorvon SD (ed.). *Handbook of Epilepsy Treatment: Forms, Causes and Therapy in Children and Adults*, 2nd edn. Oxford: Wiley-Blackwell; 2005.

Table 2.4 Clinical overview of the most common forms of generalized epilepsy

Epilepsy	Peak age of onset	Seizure type (less frequent)	Induction by photostimulation/ hyperventilation	Antiepileptic drug monotherapy	Neurological deficit	Prognosis
Idiopathic generalized epilepsy						
Juvenile myoclonic epilepsy	12–18 years	Myoclonic (tonic–clonic, absence)	Yes/No	Valproate Topiramate Lamotrigine	None	Good, requires lifelong treatment
Childhood absence epilepsy	6–7 years	Absence (tonic–clonic)	No/Yes	Valproate Ethosuximide Lamotrigine	None	Good, rapid remission with treatment
Juvenile absence epilepsy	10–12 years	Absence (tonic–clonic)	Yes/No	Valproate Ethosuximide Lamotrigine	None	Good, requires lifelong treatment
Epilepsy with myoclonic absence	≈7 years	Myoclonic absence (tonic–clonic)	No/Yes	Valproate Ethosuximide Lamotrigine	25% develop intellectual and developmental disabilities	50% remission, progression to Lennox–Gastaut possible
Epilepsy with *grand mal* on awakening	15–20 years	Generalized tonic–clonic	Yes/Yes	Phenobarbital Primidone Valproate	None	Good, requires lifelong treatment
Benign familial neonatal convulsions	2–15 days	Tonic Clonic	No/No	Phenobarbital Phenytoin Valproate	None	Good, 10% develop chronic epilepsy
Benign myoclonic epilepsy of infancy	4 months–3 years	Myoclonic	Yes/No	Valproate Benzodiazepines	None, if treatment started early	Good, discontinuation of treatment after 2–3 years
Symptomatic/ cryptogenic generalized epilepsies						
West syndrome	4–6 months	Infantile spasm	No/No	Adrenocorticotrophic hormone	Intellectual developmental delay	Variable, increased risk for chronic epilepsy

Table 2.4 (continued)

Lennox–Gastaut syndrome	1–7 years	Atypical absence Myoclonic Tonic Tonic–clonic	No/No	Valproate	Learning disability	Invariably difficult to achieve good seizure control, neurological deficit remains
Landau–Kleffner syndrome	2–7 years	Eye deviation Automatisms 2° generalization	No/No	Valproate Benzodiazepines	Intellectual, especially speech disturbance	Seizures, behavioural pychomotor disturbances often seen

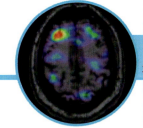
Chapter 3

Frontal Lobe Epilepsy

Introduction

The frontal lobe is the most frequent site of focal epilepsy within the extra-temporal regions. Based on this definition the onset of epilepsy is focal and not generalized and surgical resection of an epileptogenic zone in the frontal lobe would result in a surgical cure.

In patients who have medically intractable epilepsy who present to epilepsy surgical centres, approximately 10–20% of them can be expected to have frontal lobe epilepsy; however, the actual prevalence of frontal lobe epilepsy in the general population may be significantly larger. The actual prevalence is difficult to ascertain due to the difficulty in localizing the epileptogenic zone in many of these cases. Many clinical features of the seizures that are considered typical for frontal lobe epilepsy might actually have an onset outside the frontal lobe. Therefore, typical seizures associated with frontal lobe epilepsy can arise from regions such as the posterior cingulate, lateral temporal, and parietal as well as the occipital lobe. In some types of seizures particular parts of the frontal lobe can be speculated as the onset of the seizures based on the description of them. In cases when there is no lesion seen on imaging studies the exact localization for seizure onset can be difficult. In situations when the seizures are medically intractable, testing for the localization of the seizure onset zone is done to evaluate the potential for epilepsy surgery. However, when the seizures are under good control the localization of the seizure onset may be more speculative making the exact prevalence of frontal lobe epilepsy more difficult to ascertain.

Seizures that originate from the lateral frontal and basal frontal cortices will be discussed in this chapter. The seizures originating from mesial frontal cortices will be considered in another chapter as they have particular characteristics that warrant more attention. Also discussed in a separate chapter will be the topic of opercular/insular lobe epilepsy not covered here.

Anatomy of the frontal lobe

The anatomical boundaries of the frontal lobe (**3.1**) are demarcated posteriorly by the central sulcus of Rolando, mesially by the interhemispheric fissure, and inferiorly by the Sylvian fissure. The frontal lobe includes approximately one-third of the entire cortical surface of the brain. It is separated from the temporal lobe by the Sylvian fissure; medially it is separated from the limbic lobe by the cingulated gyrus; and separated from the parietal lobe by a line drawn from the marginal end of the central sulcus to the cingulate sulcus at the mesial border and by the central sulcus on the lateral border. The basal portion of the orbital surface is entirely in the frontal lobe. The lateral convexity contains the several gyri with the least variable gyral anatomy, including the precentral gyrus, superior, middle and inferior frontal gyrus. The medial aspect containing the cingulate gyrus and the basal surface is divided into gyrus rectus, as well as the medial and lateral orbital gyrus. The gyrus rectus is the medial most gyrus on the basal surface bordered by the olfactory sulcus on its lateral boundary.

Functional anatomy

The main functional regions of the cortex were defined by stimulation studies in the human and primate brain. They can be divided into primary motor areas, supplementary motor area (see Chapter 4 on Supplementary sensimotor

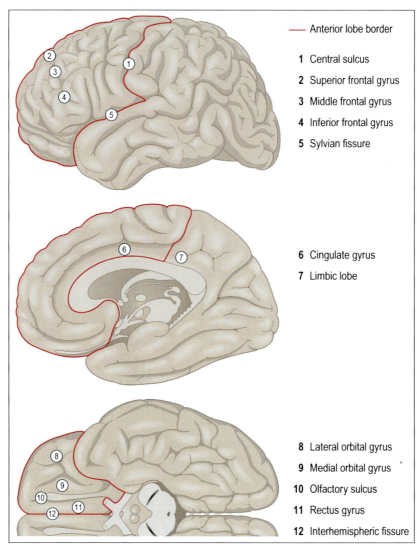

- —— Anterior lobe border

1 Central sulcus

2 Superior frontal gyrus

3 Middle frontal gyrus

4 Inferior frontal gyrus

5 Sylvian fissure

6 Cingulate gyrus

7 Limbic lobe

8 Lateral orbital gyrus

9 Medial orbital gyrus

10 Olfactory sulcus

11 Rectus gyrus

12 Interhemispheric fissure

3.1 The anatomical boundaries of the frontal lobe.

epilepsy), frontal eye field, frontal language areas (Broca's area), negative motor areas, prefrontal cortex, and orbitofrontal and anterior medial areas (see *Table 3.1*).

The primary motor areas include the posterior parts of the superior, middle and inferior frontal gyri and receive inputs from various sensorimotor regions. The main efferent output is the corticospinal tracts. This region is, as are many regions of the cortex, somatotopically organized. The frontal eye fields are located in the posterior part of the middle frontal gyrus in an area that immediately borders the primary motor cortex. Its main afferent input is from the occipital cortex and dorsal thalamus with its output projections to the preoccipital cortex and superior colliculus. The frontal language centre or Broca's area is located in the region of

the pars operculare and triangulare in the dominant frontal lobe. It is thought to have reciprocal connections to the receptive language centre located in the posterior part of the dominant temporal lobe (Wernecke's area). Also, this region has connections to the primary tongue and laryngeal motor regions as well as the auditory cortex (Heschel's gyrus) in the middle part of the dominant superior temporal gyrus as well as many other regions of the brain. The negative motor is found in the posterior part of the inferior frontal gyrus just in front of the primary motor cortex as well as in posterior aspect of the mesial frontal gyrus, which is almost continuous with the supplementary motor area in this region. The functional properties of the premotor cortex and orbitofrontal areas are less clearly defined. They include functions involved in

Table 3.1 Anatomy of the frontal lobe

Regions	Areas of cortex	Afferents	Efferents
Primary motor area	Posterior parts of the superior Middle and inferior frontal gyri	Sensorimotor regions	Corticospinal tracts
Frontal language area (Broca's area)	Pars operculare and triangulare	Posterior part of temporal lobe (Wernicke's area)	Tongue and larynx motor, Wernicke's area
Frontal eye field	Posterior part of the middle frontal gyrus bordering on primary motor cortex	Occipital cortex dorsal thalamus	Preoccipital cortex superior colliculus
Negative motor areas	Posterior part of inferior frontal gyrus and posterior mesial superior frontal gyrus	Prefrontal areas	No direct connections to spinal cord or primary motor areas

executive function, such as working memory and processing of sensory inputs of various modalities.

Seizure semiology

The cortical areas involved in the production of the seizure, the symptomatogenic zone, will determine the clinical manifestation of the seizure, i.e. seizure semiology. The knowledge of the initial symptomatogenic zone based on a patient's clinical description of the seizure may often give some information on the localization of the region, where the epilepsy arises from or the epileptogenic zone. However, there are different regions of the cortex that can produce the same clinical manifestation of a seizure, as so many times the sensitivity of the seizure semiology to locate the epileptogenic zone is poor. Another issue to keep in mind is that the initial manifestation of the seizure might reflect propagation patterns of the seizure and not information on the epileptogenic zone, particularly as there are large regions of the cortex that are 'silent' in that when stimulated do not give rise to any clinical manifestations (*Table 3.2*).

Table 3.2 Seizure semiology of the frontal lobe

Symptogenic zones	Seizure type in the frontal lobe
Primary motor cortex	Focal clonic seizures (preserved consciousness) Aura of 'tightening of body parts' Generalized tonic–clonic seizure
Frontal eye field	Head and or eye versive seizures
Anterior cingulate	Hypermotor seizures/ complex motor seizures
Frontopolar	Hypermotor seizures/ complex motor seizures
Frontal language area	Aphasic seizure
Negative motor area	Akinetic seizure

Seizures classified according to the semiological classification that can be seen in frontal lobe epilepsy are complex motor seizures. These seizures are defined as presenting with a variety of semipurposeful movements. At times they can involve more proximal musculature and are further classified as hypermotor seizures. The types of motor activity can include thrashing movements, and bicycling leg movements. The movements can be quite striking and often appear violent. These seizures tend to occur more often out of sleep. Other types of seizures include simple motor seizures originating from the primary motor cortex presenting as focal motor seizures affecting the contralateral limb of the facial muscles. These seizures can often occur in the presence of preserved awareness. Seizures arising from negative motor regions can present as a loss of tone or akinetic seizure. Seizures arising from frontal language areas can lead to a loss of speech with preserved awareness, which are called aphasic seizures. The frontal eye fields when involved in a seizure can lead to eye and or head versive movements (strong movements to the contralateral side). A variety of auras can also be seen in frontal lobe epilepsy; however, they are not of strong localization value. These auras include such descriptions as cephalic auras, abdominal auras and whole body sensations. Other descriptions such as 'racing thoughts' or a feeling of stiffening of a limb can also be seen in frontal lobe epilepsy.

Electroencephalography in frontal lobe epilepsy

Electroencephalography (EEG) findings during periods of time when no seizure is occurring in a patient, termed interictal EEG, can often be normal without any evidence of interictal epileptiform activity in up to 40% of patients. Epileptiform spike activity in frontal lobe epilepsy may not appear focal or restricted to the frontal lobe. Often spikes can appear lateralized to one hemisphere or even generalized. In some instances a leading spike can be seen preceding a more diffuse or generalized spike, which is termed secondary bilateral synchrony. When this finding is recognized it can indicate focal epilepsy as opposed to generalized epilepsy (see *case 1*).

When focal epileptiform spikes are seen, they are more likely to occur in the lateral frontal cortex and may be seen in about 50% of these cases. In the absence of a magnetic resonance imaging (MRI) lesion, focal epileptiform activity can often give some guidance for further testing or suggestions to specific modalities to further elucidate the epileptogenic zone.

EEG identified activity seen during a seizure, or ictal EEG, can vary in its utility in localization or even lateralizing the epilepsy (see *case 2*). At times, an electromyography artefact obscures the EEG so that no clear information is obtainable. This can be seen in 20% of the cases. At other times a more diffuse pattern can be seen but again not lending any further localization value. Localizable ictal EEG patterns are described in only 30–40% of cases with frontal lobe epilepsy. At times when the surface EEG shows a diffuse pattern an invasive EEG recording with subdural arrays can provide a more localized seizure onset. Focal scalp ictal onset patterns often consist of low amplitude fast activity, occasionally high amplitude spike or polyspike activity, or a leading focal spike/transient prior to more diffuse changes seen on EEG (see *case 3*).

Neuroimaging

Imaging has become the cornerstone in the evaluation of patients with epilepsy. This is particularly so in patients with medically intractable seizures. Imaging is used to address whether there is a lesion to accompany an epilepsy syndrome that is consistent in location with the clinical manifestations. Patients with lesional epilepsy have a significantly higher chance for success if they proceed to epilepsy surgery compared with those who are non-lesional. MRI has become the standard radiological tool in detecting lesions in patients with epilepsy. Various sequences such as modified T1-, T2- and proton density images have improved the ability to resolve epileptic lesions. In particular, high-resolution T1-weighted images and fluid-attenuated inversion recovery imaging has greatly improved the capability of imaging lesions on MRI. In some patients who have difficulty with claustrophobia or who are extremely overweight, sedation or an open MRI scanner may be required. On occasion when MRI is not available or if there is a question of a calcification or haemorrhagic quality to the lesion, computerized tomography might be helpful.

Positron emission tomography has been used to evaluate areas of hypometabolism that may give indirect evidence for the epileptogenic region (**3.2**). This area of hypometabolism often overestimates the region of epileptogenicity and often also incorporates the functional deficit zone. Single photon emission computed tomography (SPECT) imaging visualizes regional blood flow changes usually evaluated during the ictal state. This along with co-localization with MRI images may give some added information, particularly in MRI normal subjects (see *case 2*, **CS 2.4**).

Aetiology

A variety of aetiologies can be seen in patients with frontal lobe epilepsy. About 20–30% of one series of patients with frontal lobe epilepsy had neoplastic lesions. Not all patients with tumours develop seizures. However, many older patients do develop them. Also if tumours involve the grey matter they have a higher chance of developing seizures as are tumours in the central region of the brain. In terms of types of tumours

from highest to lowest prevalence of seizures are low-grade astrocytoma, mixed gliomas and gangliogliomas. On the other hand glioblastoma, metastases and meningiomas have a lower chance for seizures, although seizures are known to occur in this setting as well (see *case 4*).

Cortical dysplasia (the term used for malformations of the cortex that result from aberrant neuronal migration) is a common aetiology seen in surgical series of frontal lobe epilepsy. In one series the frequency of cortical dysplasia was as high as 58% based on surgical pathology. These patients also appear to have more intrinsic epileptogenicity than ganglioglioma. The reason for this is not clear but may be due to an overexpression of a subtype of the *N*-methyl-D-aspartic acid receptor associated with increased excitability (see *Table 3.3*).

Cerebral vascular malformations are developmental vascular lesions in the central nervous system. Only about 5% of these lesions are thought to give rise to epilepsy. These vascular malformations can be divided into arteriovascular malformations, cavernous angiomas, venous malformations and telangiectasias. They are found in patients with frontal lobe epilepsy in 6–14% of cases.

Encephalomalacia as a result of head trauma can lead to epilepsy and at times medically intractable epilepsy. The history of head injury, therefore, is an important risk factor in the later development of epilepsy. Frontal pole and basal frontal regions are particularly at risk to injury during head trauma and are common locations for signs of encephalomalacia. Other types of head trauma such as penetrating injuries and depressed skull fractures also are considered significant for the later development of epilepsy (see *case 4*).

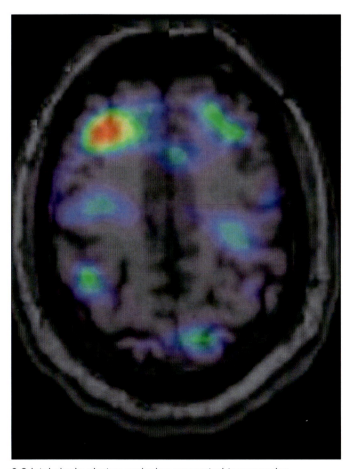

3.2 Ictal single photon emission computed tomography showing findings of seizure onset in the right frontocentral region. Based on these findings the assessment for epilepsy surgery recommended further evaluation using subdural electrodes covering the right lateral convexity, including the right frontocentral region.

Table 3.3 Aetiologies seen in seven surgical series of frontal lobe epilepsy

Aetiology	No. of patients
Tumour	50%
Cortical dysplasia	19%
Gliosis	11%
Encephalomalacia	10%
Vascular malformation	10%

Case studies

Case 1

A 21-year-old right-handed man had seizures that began at 18 years of age. They consisted of generalized motor seizures that occurred out of sleep. His seizures are currently well controlled on medications. His EEG and imaging findings are seen in **CS 1.1–1.3**.

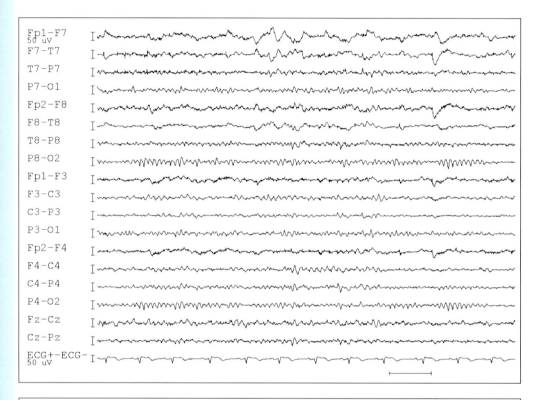

CS 1.1 Intermittent slowing is seen over the left frontotemporal regions. This signifies an area of dysfunction in this area. There is, however, no epileptiform activity, which is not uncommon in patients with frontal lobe epilepsy.

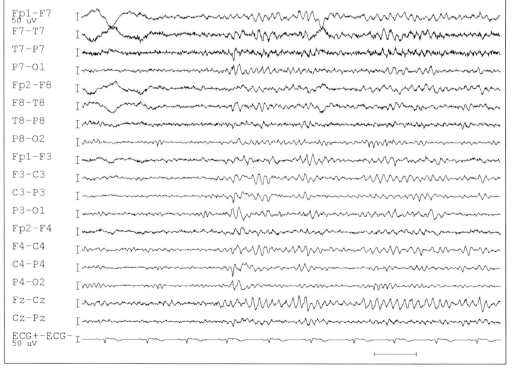

CS 1.2 Generalized slowing is seen higher over the left frontal region. This finding is significantly more subtle. There is clearly visualized theta range slowing seen diffusely; on closer examination, however, it can be appreciated that the slowing is more prominent over the left hemisphere than on the right. More generalized and lateralized interictal findings of slowing can be seen as a feature of frontal dysfunction.

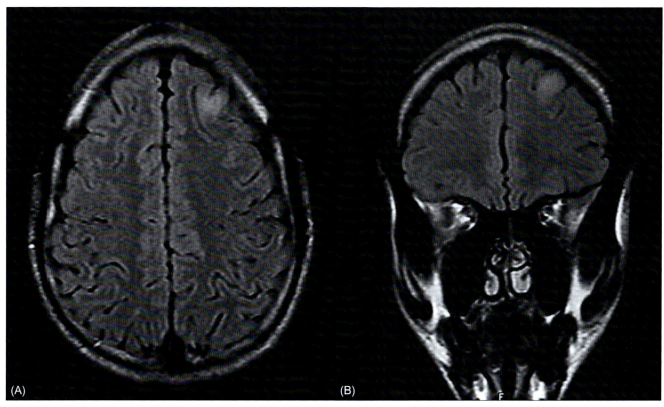

CS 1.3 Fluid-attenuated inversion recovery magnetic resonance images showing an increase in signal involving the anterior portion of the left middle frontal gyrus. These results are likely supportive of cortical dysplasia or a low-grade glioma/dysembryoplastic neuroepithelial tumour. These findings together suggest that the patient has left frontal lobe epilepsy; however, he is under good medical control. He has yearly imaging of this lesion without any significant change in the imaging findings.

Case 2

This is a 42-year-old right-handed man whose seizures began at the age of 8 years. His seizures are described by an aura, which consists of a feeling of 'being stuck in the moment and unable to think about anything else'. He begins to hyperventilate but he is not aware of this part of the seizure. Observers state that he makes repetitive movements, loud noises and kicking. During this part of the seizure he is usually unresponsive but has responded to some questions with no recollection. He has four to six seizures per month and has failed multiple different anticonvulsant medications. He has a normal MRI scan of the brain. His EEG (interictal/ictal) and ictal SPECT scans are seen in **CS 2.1–2.4**.

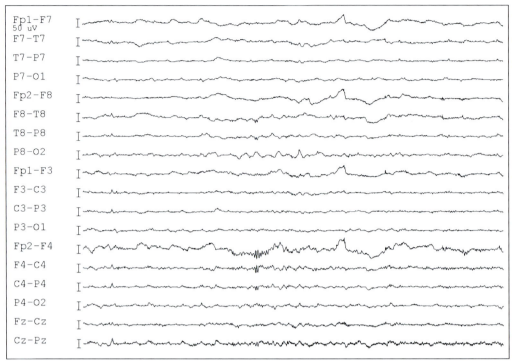

CS 2.1 Asymmetry increased spindles over the right frontocentral region.

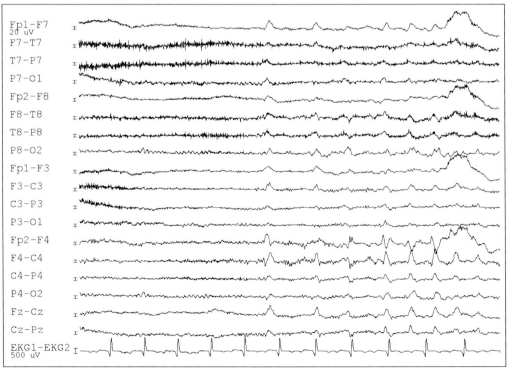

CS 2.2 Frequent interictal epileptiform activity is seen over the right frontocentral region resembling a periodic lateralized epileptiform discharge-like pattern.

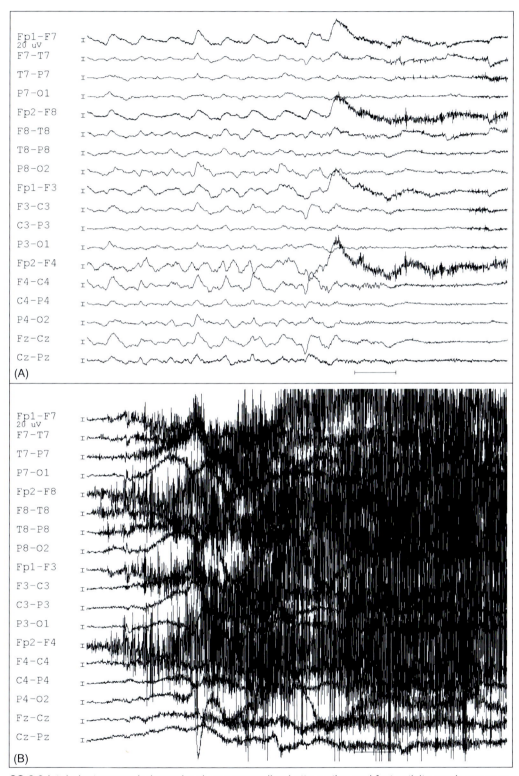

CS 2.3 Ictal electroencephalography shows generalized attenuation and fast activity maximum over the right frontocentral region.

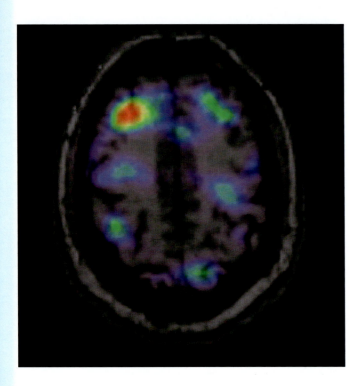

CS 2.4 Ictal single photon emission computed tomography shows findings of seizure onset in the right frontocentral region. Based on these findings the assessment for epilepsy surgery recommended further evaluation with invasive electrodes using subdural electrodes covering the right lateral convexity, including the right frontocentral region.

Case 3 (see opposite)

This is a 46-year-old right-handed woman whose seizures began at the age of 13 years. Her seizures consist of a guttural sound with complaints that her throat is tightening and she has effortful speech, which leads to a contraction of the right side of her face followed by a generalized clonic seizure. Her MRI scan is within normal limits (**CS 3.1–3.6**).

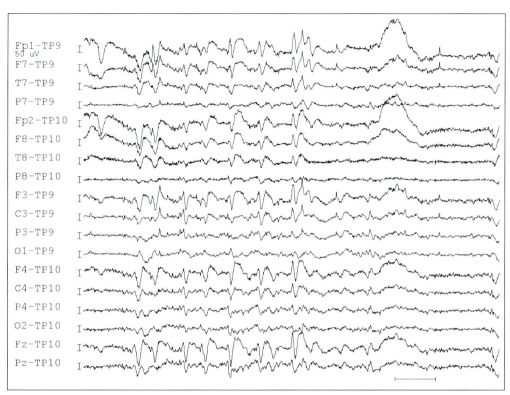

CS 3.1 A generalized spike–wave complex is seen. This sort of interictal electroencephalography finding would be consistent with a patient with generalized epilepsy. However, occasionally, they can also be seen in cases of frontal lobe epilepsy.

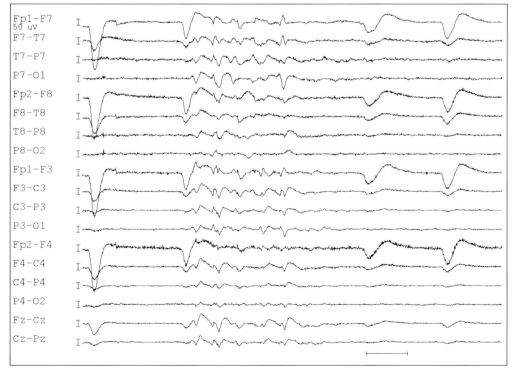

CS 3.2 The same patient's electroencephalography patterns show some generalized spike–wave complex that are seen more maximally over the left hemisphere.

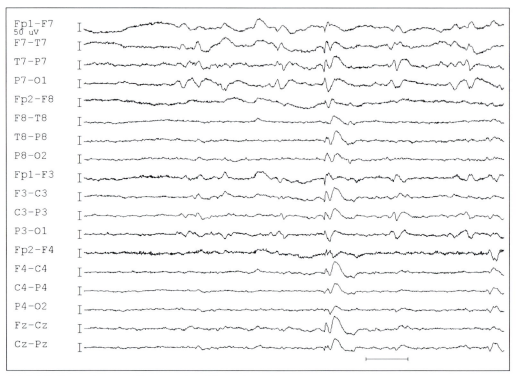

CS 3.3 Spike and wave with secondary bilateral synchrony.

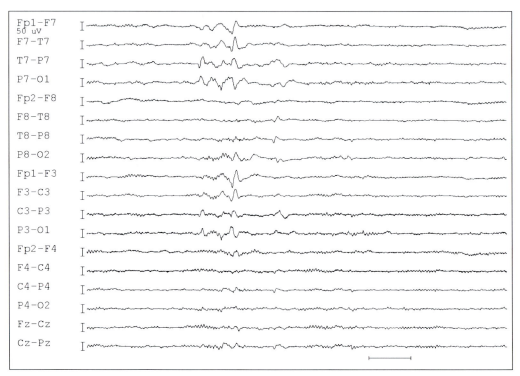

CS 3.4 Left parietal spike following a more diffuse pattern over the left hemisphere.

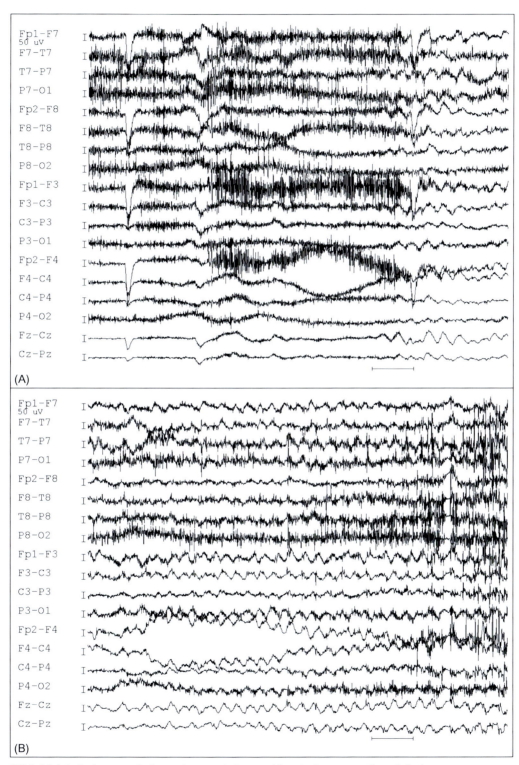

CS 3.5 Ictal electroencephalography onset obscured by electromyography artefacts.

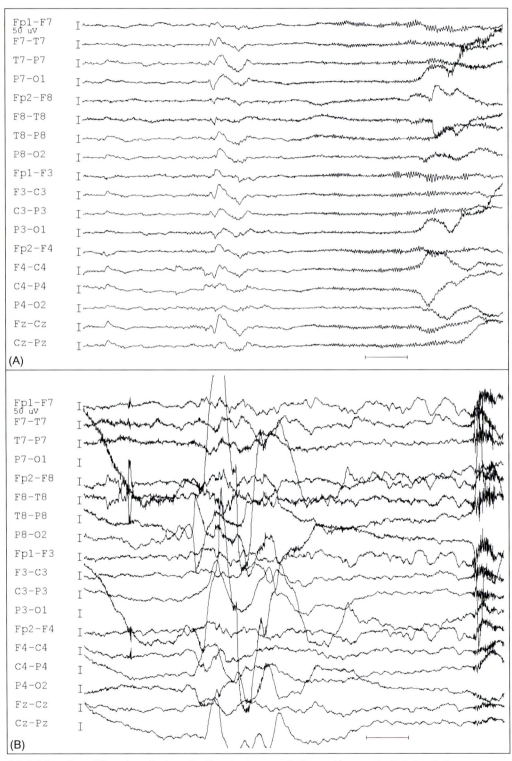

CS 3.6 Leading diffuse transient marks the electroencephalographic onset of ictal activity.

Case 4

A 59-year-old right-handed woman had presented 1 month previously with an episode of left facial and arm tightness that evolved into an inability to speak following which she developed urine and bowel incontinence. She remained conscious throughout the episode. The episode lasted for several minutes. She underwent debulking of a right frontal glioblastoma and underwent chemotherapy and radiotherapy. She was noted to have further seizures and required intubation. An EEG was obtained to rule out further seizures (**CS 4.1–4.3**).

Conclusions

The term frontal lobe epilepsy consists of a variety of different disease entities. Various features of these patients, including seizure semiology, imaging findings and EEG patterns may suggest this diagnosis. Non-lesional cases of frontal lobe epilepsy and generalized features on the EEG pose difficulties in diagnosis.

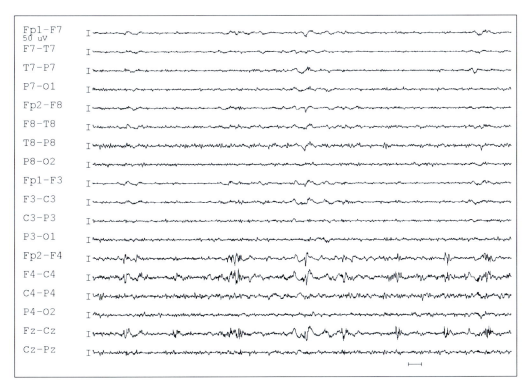

CS 4.1 Periodic lateralized epileptiform discharges are seen in the right frontocentral region in a patient with a right frontal glioblastoma. Some of the sharp waves have a polyspike morphology that can be seen in patients with tumours.

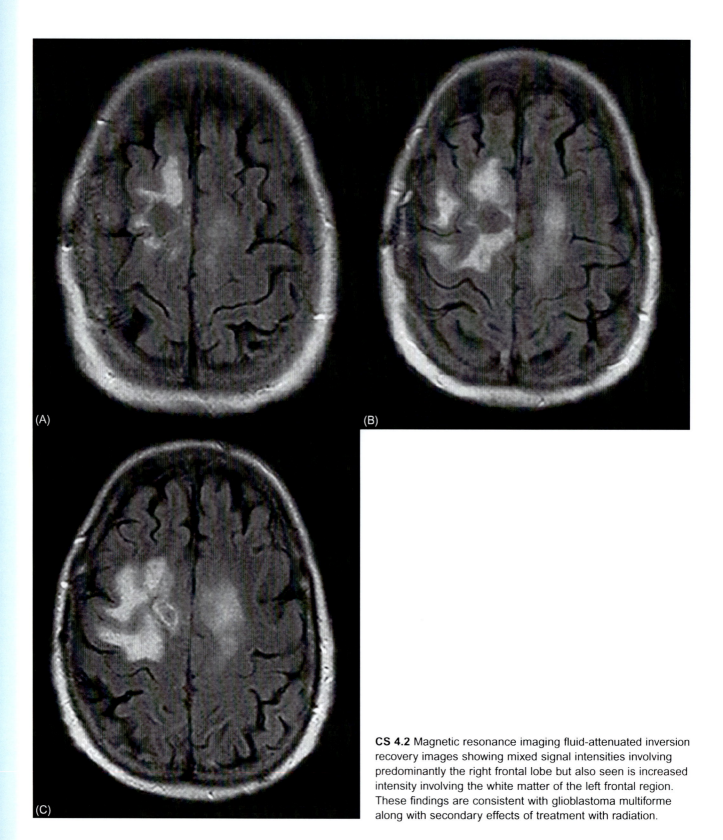

(A)

(B)

(C)

CS 4.2 Magnetic resonance imaging fluid-attenuated inversion recovery images showing mixed signal intensities involving predominantly the right frontal lobe but also seen is increased intensity involving the white matter of the left frontal region. These findings are consistent with glioblastoma multiforme along with secondary effects of treatment with radiation.

Further reading

Garcia PA, Laxar KD. Lateral frontal lobe epilepsies. In: Lüders HO, Comair Y, eds. *Epilepsy Surgery*. Philadephia: Lippincott Williams & Wilkins; 2001: 111–118.

Holthausen H, Hoppe M. Hypermotor seizures. In: Lüders HO, Noachtar S, eds. *Epileptic Seizures: Pathophysiology and Clinical Semiology*. New York: Churchill Livingstone; 2000: 439–48.

Kellinghaus C, Lüders HO. Frontal lobe epilepsy. *Epileptic Disord* 2004; **6**: 223–39.

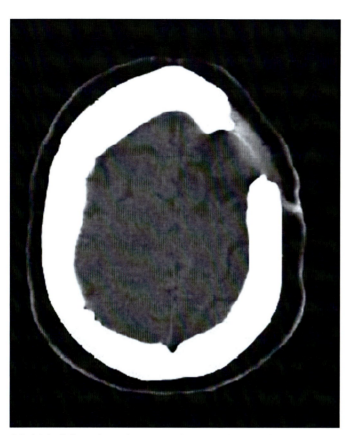

CS 4.3 Left frontal craniotomy and encephalomalacia in a patient with medically intractable focal epilepsy with several admissions for status epilepticus. The lesion is demonstrated by computed tomography as opposed to magnetic resonance imaging in this extremely overweight individual.

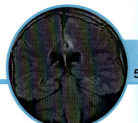

Chapter 4

Supplementary Sensorimotor Epilepsy

Introduction

As discussed in Chapter 3, frontal lobe epilepsy presents a diagnostic and therapeutic challenge to clinicians, particularly as it refers to patients with medically refractory seizures arising from the frontal lobe. There is a bizarre and unfamiliar semiology that can present with frontal lobe epilepsy—at times this can bring into question whether the patient in fact has epilepsy or psychogenic seizures. Seizures arising from the mesial frontal lobe or within the supplementary sensorimotor area (SSMA) are of particular interest because patients may be well aware of their surroundings during what appears to be a generalized motor seizure. Typically, one would expect consciousness to be impaired during such a seizure but in cases of SSMA seizures, consciousness may be retained. Seizures arising from areas near or adjacent to the SSMA, such as the mesial frontal lobe, often propagate quickly to the SSMA, displaying SSMA seizure semiology; therefore, a minority of these patients with SSMA seizures actually have supplementary sensorimotor epilepsy (SSME). SSME is rare, with an incidence among epileptics undergoing video-electroencephalography (video-EEG) monitoring to be as low as 2.0%. It can be lesional or non-lesional with a broad array of aetiologies, including cortical dysplasia, encephalomalcia and idiopathic aetiologies. It usually presents with ambiguous EEG abnormalities, if with any, and with scalp EEG it is difficult to correctly localize. In cases of medically refractory SSME, particularly those associated with a lesion a surgical resection may yield a good outcome with only a transient neurological deficit. However, proper identification of the epileptogenic zone is of prime importance as in all cases of surgical treatment for epilepsy, but the recognition of involvement of the SSMA region might yield clues as to its correct location. Astute and careful clinical practice is required to correctly identify and treat this epilepsy, which can be so easily mistaken for another syndrome.

Anatomy of the supplementary sensorimotor area

Classically the frontal motor cortex is divided functionally into the primary, premotor, and supplementary motor regions. The SSMA occupies the medial and superolateral portion of Brodmann's area 6. It represents the body topographically, with the head located in the anterior portion and the legs and the feet in the posterior part, adjacent to Brodmann's area 4. It has complex reciprocal connections with the lateral frontal cortex. The corpus callosum also joins homotopic areas of both the SSMA on both hemispheres. Other afferents include input from the basal ganglia (globus pallidus and pars reticularis of substantia nigra). It receives both proprioceptive and cutaneous afferents from the ventral posterosuperior nucleus and the ventral posterolateral nucleus of the thalamus.

Cortical stimulation elicits more complex motor responses in the SSMA when compared with the primary motor cortex with a greater threshold for responses to electrical stimulation. Corticospinal projections from the SSMA terminate principally on spinal interneurons and not directly on lower motor neurons. It should also be noted that SSMA afferents drive upper motor neurons in the primary motor cortex (**4.1**).

Seizure semiology

Seizures arising from the SSMA have a distinctive ictal semiology that may allow a provisional diagnosis to be made on

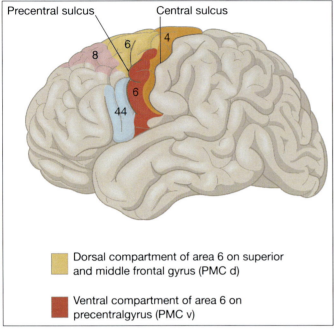

4.1 Distribution of Brodmann's agranular and dysgranular cytoarchitectonic areas 4, 6, 8, and 44 on the precentral frontal gyri. Colours designate the different cytoarchitectonic areas and subdivide area 6 into a ventral compartment, which lies in the precentral gyrus and a dorsal part, covering the superior and middle frontal gyri. Area 8 is also known as the frontal eye field and is responsible for eye movements, sending projections to the lateral gaze centre in the paramedium pontine reticular formation. Area 44 is also known as Broca's area and is responsible for the motor aspects of speech, sending projections to Wernicke's area via the arcuate fasiculus. CS, central sulcus; PCS, precentral sulcus.

review of clinical history alone (*Table 4.1*). Seizures have been noted to be extremely brief, lasting between 10 and 40 seconds only. They usually begin abruptly without warning and manifest directly with motor phenomena. Asymmetric posturing involving the extremities bilaterally usually marks the onset. Unilateral tonic motor activity may also occur, although it is not as frequent. The shoulders are usually elevated and the arms abducted with some flexion of the elbows. The lower limbs may also show abducted hips with knees either extended or semi-flexed. It has been reported that all four extremities are tonically postured, however, asymmetrically. During the ictal semiology consciousness may be preserved, so that during the tonic phase of this seizure the patient may appear to attempt to move body position, such as trying to sit up straight or may display writhing truncal movements. Orofacial and gestural automatisms are absent; however,

patients may display coarse, uncoordinated movements of their tonically postured limbs. Bizarrely, asynchronous use of all four limbs with preservation of consciousness may lead to the misdiagnosis of psychogenic seizures, observing tonically abducted arms combined with open eyes, predominant nocturnal occurrence and the brevity of the seizure is useful in distinguishing a SSMA seizure from a psychogenic seizure.

During the tonic phase of the seizure, speech arrest occurs slightly more frequently than vocalization. Vocalizations take the form of the patient crying out or moaning loudly and intelligible speech is extremely rare. Some vocalizations may be due to the involuntary contraction of the diaphragm or the laryngeal muscles, and, in others, they appear to be emotional responses to their awareness of seizure onset. The tonic phase is then followed by a clonic phase during which one or more extremity move in a rhythmic or clonic manner. Versive head movements often occur prior to secondary generalization and serve as a reliable lateralizing sign in this setting, lateralizing to the contralateral hemisphere. Seizures tend to occur in clusters, and as many as five to 20 per day have been observed in patients with intractable SSMA epilepsy and thus can be very disabling.

Electroencephalography in supplementary sensorimotor epilepsy

Unfortunately, scalp EEG findings are usually of little localizing value. If midline electrodes are not placed, epileptiform discharges may be missed. Sharp waves are usually found near or adjacent to the midline, and, if only occurring during sleep, it may be difficult to distinguish them from normal sleep transients. It should be noted, however, that polyspikes and spikes followed by a prominent aftergoing slow wave are suggestive of epileptiform activity. In children in whom vertex waves tend to have a particularly sharp morphology, the correct identification of SSMA epileptic discharges may be difficult. Careful examination of the symmetry of the electrical field discharges may be helpful, noting that normal sleep structures have symmetric electrical fields.

The phenomena 'paradoxic lateralization' occurs often in SSMA epilepsy further complicating the localization of the epileptogenic zone. If a spike is generated in the interhemispheric fissure, a transverse or oblique dipole will be created, so that a right hemispheric focus adjacent to the

Table 4.1 Most prominent semiologies in supplementary sensorimotor area (SSMA) seizures and psychogenic seizures that lead to confusion between these two distinct pathologies

Common seizure semiology

SSMA	Psychogenic
Duration very short: 10–40 seconds	Duration longer: >40 seconds
Predominantly during sleep	Predominantly in awake state
Consciousness retained	Consciousness retained
Tonic posturing: abduction of upper extremities	Tonic posturing: no abduction of upper extremities
Opisthotonic posturing: neck only	Opisthotonic posturing: neck and trunk
Versive head movement before secondary generalization	No lateralizing semiology
Thrashing movements stereotypic entire body legs only more frequent mimicking kicking	Thrashing movements unpredictable entire body head and neck only more frequent
Ends abruptly: without postictal confusion	Ends abruptly: without postictal confusion

midline might produce an electrical maximum over the left hemisphere near the midline.

The prominent motor activity from the onset of the seizure can make the ictal EEG recordings difficult to interpret, as they are often rendered useless due to prominent electromyographic and movement artefact that obscures the EEG recording. Characteristic findings include an initial high-amplitude slow wave transient or a midline sharp wave followed by midline fast activity. Low-voltage fast activity often evolves into generalized rhythmic theta slowing. Slow activity or low-voltage fast activity can localize to the vertex or more diffusely, although lateralizing information is usually minimal. Sometimes there is no observable EEG change found during a SSMA seizure (in approximately 6% of cases); however, it should not be prematurely presumed that the patient has psychogenic seizures and further studies should performed. Invasive EEG studies, usually consisting of strategically placed subdural grids or stereo-EEG depth electrodes, are more fruitful and can be utilized in SSMA epilepsy cases preceding surgical treatment.

Neuroimaging

As with other modalities used to localize an epileptic lesion, SSMA epilepsy is often elusive to standard neuroimaging techniques. Studies have shown conventional magnetic resonance imaging (MRI) to yield fewer abnormalities in SSMA epilepsy in comparison with other types of focal epilepsy. MRI has been shown to reliably identify abnormalities such as ischemic insults, encephalomalacia, neoplasms and other lesions. It is of value to note that those patients with SSMA epilepsy, who post-resection were shown with histological studies to have cortical dysplasia, often displayed no abnormality on MRI.

Ictal single photon emission computed tomography (SPECT) has been shown to be useful in lateralizing SSMA epilepsy correctly. It is important, however, to inject the tracer as soon as possible due to the extremely short duration of the seizure. Injections given 10–15 s after ictal onset are thought to be useless due to the rapid propagation of epileptic discharges. An optimal injection time less than 5 s after ictal onset is thought to be useful for the lateralization of SSMA epilepsy.

Positron emission tomography scans may occasionally be of benefit in SSMA epilepsy, in demonstrating areas of hypometabolism. However, these areas of hypometabolism may not be confined to the SSMA and can reflect the ictal spread of epileptic discharges and the motor phenomena seen during the seizure.

Aetiology

SSMA epilepsy can arise from a wide variety of aetiologies. It is unusual, however, for instance, for an ischaemic insult to occur directly at this very specific and anatomically quite small area of cortex. Patients tend to have suffered from insults that have a more global effect on the cortex such as encephalitis, head trauma or congenital malformations. SSMA epilepsy may frequently present as non-lesional epilepsy in neuroimaging studies; many such patients who undergo surgery are found to have cortical dysplasia after histopathological studies have been performed.

Case studies

Case 1

The patient presented 5 years after the initial onset of her seizures at age 12. They started with an aura comprising of a tingling or numb sensation all over her body followed by loss of awareness and generalized tonic posturing lasting 20–40 seconds. On occasion these were secondarily generalized seizures. EEG monitoring located the ictal onset to the central region with ictal SPECT studies further localizing it to the left frontoparietel region. Neuroimaging studies showed an area of dysplasia over the anterior mesial frontal region. With these findings an invasive evaluation was performed, placing subdural grids over the central region as well as covering the anterior and posterior left frontal lobe. Subsequent recordings localized the seizure onset zone to the left SSMA. The risks and benefits of a left SSMA resection were discussed with the patient. Before resection of this area, extensive intraoperative cortical mapping was done, identifying the right hand and right leg areas. Cortical dysplasia was confirmed histopathologically (**CS 1.1**). Postoperatively, as expected, she manifested a SSMA syndrome consisting of an initial right hemiparesis

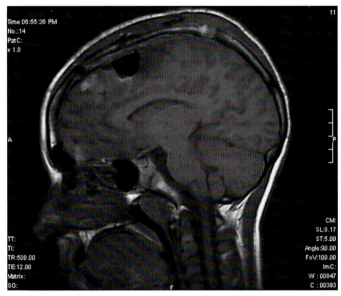

CS 1.1 A T1-weighted magnetic resonance image in the saggital plane shows, postoperatively, the resected sensorimotor area.

and difficulty in initiating speech. After restorative therapy and speech therapy, she returned to her neurological baseline and has remained seizure free.

Case 2

A 16-year-old patient presented 1 year after his first seizure. His history was significant for head trauma at 12 years of age with loss of consciousness for a brief period. His main seizure type occurred chiefly at night, consisting of stiffening of an extended right arm while the left arm was flexed; these seizures lasted approximately 30 s and could be accompanied by urinary incontinence or tongue biting. He also displayed a second seizure type that manifested initially as an epigastric aura, followed by staring and drooling that eventually evolved into oral and manual automatisms. Video-EEG monitoring localized the epilepsy to the left frontal lobe, with frequent spikes seen in the left frontal region accompanied by intermittent slowing. EEG seizures were obscured by muscle artefact; however, postictally there was diffuse slowing seen in the left hemisphere (**CS 2.1**). MR imaging showed an abnormal hypointensity involving the grey–white matter in the dorsal aspect of the left cingulate gyrus, which was felt to be suggestive of a low-grade glioma (**CS 2.2**). He underwent invasive evaluation for further, more precise, localization of the ictal onset with subdural electrode placement along the anterior and posterior aspects of the hemispheric fissure

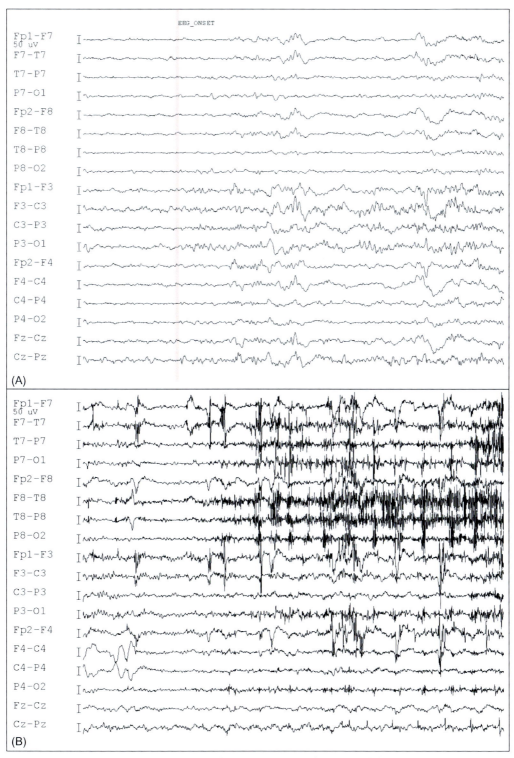

CS 2.1 Electroencephalography recordings show the start of a seizure arising from the left fronto central region as well as some left fronto central intermittent slowing. Unfortunately as the seizure progresses it is obscured by muscle artefact and cannot be further quantified.

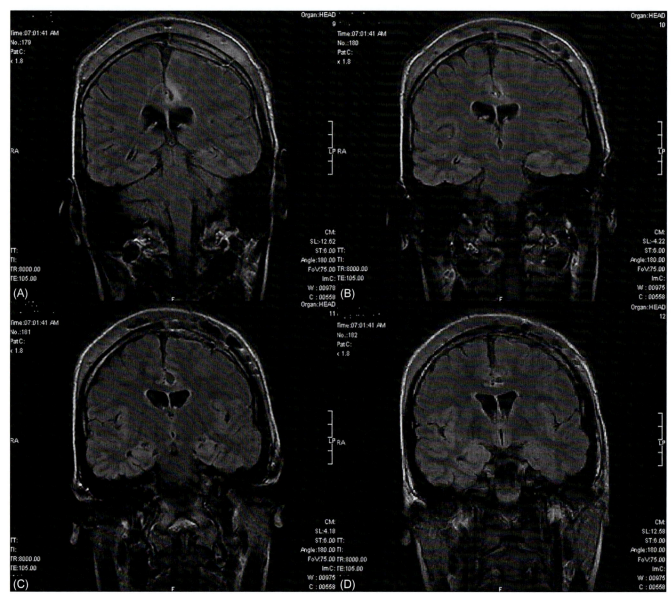

CS 2.2 T1-weighted fluid-attenuated inversion recovery magnetic resonance images in the coronal plane showing a lesion in the left supplementary sensorimotor area. This lesion was non-enhancing on T1-weighted gadolinium imaging suggestive of an astrocytoma.

as well as covering the lateral surface of the frontal lobe. A biopsy of the foot region of the left SSMA was performed, which was confirmed histopathologically as an astrocytoma. The ictal onset was confirmed to be located in the left SSMA. After discussion with the patient and parents, the left cingular gyrus was resected. Initially, postoperatively, he displayed complete right lower extremity hemiplegia, which improved to a pre-operative baseline with restorative treatment. He has remained seizure free.

Conclusions

Fortunately, SSME has a striking semiology, which in the absence of easily attainable scalp EEG and neuroimaging evidence points the physician to its probable diagnosis. The physician must take care not to mistake SSMA epilepsy for psychogenic seizures, even in the presence of retained awareness during seizures and pharmacoresistant seizures. Surgical resection is a good option for intractable SSMA epilepsy; however, it often requires extensive invasive studies to be performed for the correct localization of the epileptogenic zone and the protection of eloquent cortex during surgery.

Further reading

Ikeda A, Sato T, Ohara S, *et al.* 'Supplementary motor area (SMA) seizure' rather than 'SMA epilepsy' in optimal surgical candidates: a document of subdural mapping. *J Neurol Sci* 2002; **202**: 43–52.

Kanner AM, Morris HH, Lüders HO, *et al.* Supplementary motor seizures mimicking pseudoseizures: some clinical differences. *Neurology* 1990; **40**: 1404–7.

Laich E, Kuzniecky R, Mountz J, *et al.* Supplementary sensorimotor area epilepsy. Seizure localization, cortical propagation and subcortical activation pathways using ictal SPECT. *Brain* 1997; **120**: 855–64.

Lüders HO (ed.). *Supplementary Sensorimotor Area: Advances in Neurology*, Vol. 70. Philadelphia: Lippincott, Williams and Wilkins; 1996.

Lüders HO, Comair Y (eds). *Epilepsy Surgery.* New York: Lippincott, Williams and Wilkins; 2001.

Lüders HO, Noachtar S (eds). *Epileptic Seizures: Pathophysiology and Clinical Semiology.* New York: Saunders; 2000.

Matsumoto R, Nair D, LaPresto E, Bingaman W, Shibasaki H, Lüders HO. Functional connectivity in human cortical motor system: a cortico-cortical evoked potential study. *Brain* 2007; **130**: 181–97.

Morris HH, Dinner D, Lüders HO, Wyllie E, Kramer R. Supplementary motor seizures: clinical and electroencephalographic findings. *Neurology* 1988; **38**: 1075–82.

Schmitt JJ, Janszky J, Woermann F, Tuxhorn I, Ebner A. Laughter and the mesial and lateral premotor cortex. *Epilepsy Behav* 2006; **8**: 773–5.

Chapter 5

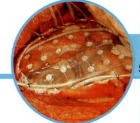

Temporal Lobe Epilepsy

Introduction

Temporal lobe epilepsy (TLE) is a type of focal epilepsy where the seizures arise from the temporal lobe and adjoining structures. TLE is the most prevalent form of focal epilepsy in adults and is the syndrome that is most successfully treated by resective surgery. TLE can be further divided into mesial (mTLE) and neocortical (nTLE). The seizures are usually characterized by manual and oral automatisms (automotor seizure) as opposed to more proximal motor automatisms (hypermotor seizure) as seen predominantly in frontal lobe epilepsy, and are often preceded by a distinctive epigastric, psychic or abdominal aura. Secondary generalized tonic–clonic seizures are also not uncommon. There can be subtle differences in seizure semiology between mTLE and nTLE that will be discussed later. Lateralizing signs during seizures are important to identify and lateralize the symptomatogenic zone in TLE. It has been reported that 78% of patients presented with lateralizing signs during seizures and with a combined positive predictive value of 94%.

Epilepsy is not a static disease and is known to progress. Hippocampal sclerosis has been recognized as one of the main aetiologies in patients with mTLE. Initially, patients with TLE can be medically controlled; however, later they may evolve to develop medically intractable seizures. It is important to diagnose mTLE as early as possible, once they become medically intractable, as disabling seizures in 80–90% of patients can be eliminated by an anteriomesial temporal lobectomy. There is evidence to suggest that early resection provides the greatest opportunity for fewer psychosocial adverse events.

Anatomy of the temporal lobe

The Sylvian sulcus separates the temporal lobe from the frontal and parietal lobes with the parahippocampal gyrus marking the medial surface. There are four longitudinally orientated gyri in the temporal lobe: (1) the superior temporal gyrus (extending to the superficial transverse temporal gyrus); (2) the middle temporal gyrus; (3) the inferior temporal gyrus located on the lateral and inferolateral surface; and (4) the occipitotemporal gyrus located on the inferior surface (5.1A,B).

The superficial transverse temporal gyrus and adjacent portions of the superior temporal gyrus receive thalamic afferent fibres from the medial geniculate nuclei, representing the primary auditory cortex (Brodmann's area 41 and part of 42) (5.1C). The neurons in this part of the cortex are organized tonotopically, mirroring the topographic map of frequency representation on the basilar membrane. The cortical connections for discerning the various elements of speech project to the adjacent temporal cortex, Wernicke's area and the posterior parietal cortex, as well as other regions. Several secondary areas surround the primary auditory cortex, each with tonotopic organization.

The pulvinar nuclei and the visual cortex influence the remaining temporal gyri (known collectively as the inferior temporal association cortex). They are involved in visual and acoustic cognition, visual discrimination and pattern perception, which can be explained by their neighbouring cortices of the posterior parietal association cortex and the occipital association cortex.

Seizure semiology

Seizures of temporal lobe origin may begin with an aura. Epigastric auras are the most frequent in TLE, described often as a 'rising sensation' beginning in the abdomen. Other

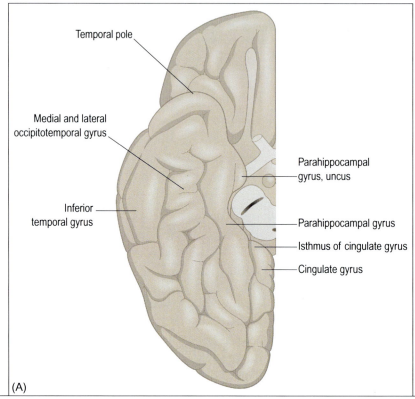

(A)

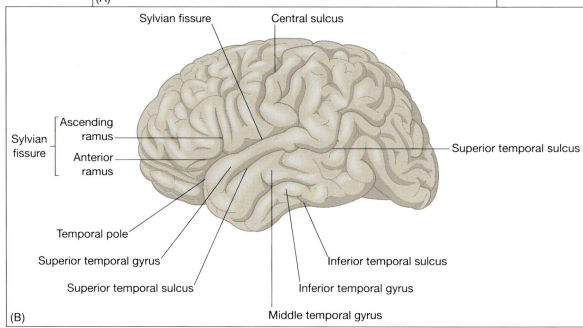

(B)

5.1 (A) Temporal gyri and sulci from the inferior aspect. (B) Lateral aspect of left lateral lobe.

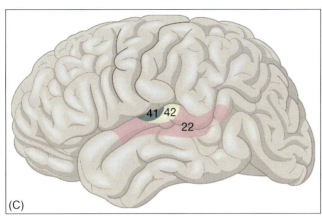

(C)

5.1 (*continued*) (C) Brodmann's cortical areas of the left temporal lobe from the lateral aspect. Area 41 represents the primary auditory cortex, area 42 the associative auditory cortex and the posterior part of area 22 represents Wernicke's area, which is responsible for the comprehension of speech.

common auras in patients with TLE include psychic, fear, auditory and olfactory auras. The occurrence of these auras gives some localization information, i.e. that they may begin in the temporal lobe but are not very helpful in lateralizing information, i.e. whether they begin in the right or left temporal lobe. Focal clonic movement has been found to lateralize the sympatogenic zone to the contralateral side of the movement, but these findings are not usually seen in the initial part of the seizure semiology in TLE. In contrast, in seizures occurring in the frontal and parietal lobes, there may be an occurrence of focal motor symptoms early in their seizure evolution.

Automatisms are a prominent feature of TLE seizures, taking many forms. Some believe unilateral motor automatisms to be of ipsilateral lateralizing value, which is most likely due to the presence of contralateral dystonic posturing masking the automatism in the contralateral limb. Oro-alimentary automatisms consisting usually of a chewing motion and lip smacking can be frequently seen in seizures of temporal lobe origin but may also occur in seizures arising outside the temporal lobe as well. Automatisms have been induced by electrical stimulation of the amygdala. Manual automatisms consist of movements involving the limbs, in which the patient appears to be fumbling, grasping, pulling at the bed sheets or manipulating an object within reach. The occurrence of motor automatisms in conjunction with dystonic posturing has been attributed to a specific primary spread of seizure discharges to subcortical brain structures and not to the

seizure onset. This progression has subsequently been shown to be more common in mTLE and has been suggested as a criterion to distinguish between mTLE and nTLE. *Table 5.1* lists common semiology for mTLE and nTLE, as well as noting differences.

Table 5.1 Common seizure semiology

Mesial TLE	Lateral TLE

Tripartite seizure pattern:
    aura
    absence
    automatism
	Tripartite seizure pattern:
	    aura
	    (absence less
	    common)
	    automatism

Aura
    visceral
    cephalic
    gustatory
    affective
    autonomic
	Aura
	    visual hallucinations
	    auditory hallucinations

Partial awareness—in early stages preserved	Partial awareness—in early stages preserved
Dystonic posturing of contralateral limb with ipsilateral automatisms	Tonic posturing or jerking more common
Speech arrest during seizures with postictal dyphasia (dominant hemisphere only)	Speech arrest during seizures with postictal dyphasia (dominant hemisphere only)

Automatisms
    oro-alimentary
    gestural
    sometimes prolonged
	Automatisms
	    oro-alimentary
	    gestural
	    sometimes prolonged

Autonomic changes common	Autonomic changes common
Postictal confusion common	Postictal confusion common
Secondary generalization infrequent	Secondary generalization more frequent

TLE, temporal lobe epilepsy.

Table 5.2

Ictal feature	Side relative to seizure onset
Reliable signs	
Unilateral dystonic posturing	Contralateral
Unilateral automatisms	Ipsilateral
Ictal speech	Non-dominant hemisphere
Postictal dysphasia	Dominant hemisphere
Forced head turning before secondary generalization (version)	Contralateral
Less reliable signs	
Head turning at onset of seizure	Ipsilateral
Ictal blinking	Ipsilateral
Ictal spitting	Ipsilateral
Ictal vomitting	Non-dominant hemisphere
Postictal nose wiping	Ipsilateral

Dystonic posturing of limbs is regarded of high lateralizing value in TLE, lateralizing to a symptomatogenic zone contralaterally. During the tonic phase of a secondary generalized tonic–clonic seizure the patient extends one elbow while flexing the other and forming what appears to be a 'figure 4 sign'—the extended elbow is contralateral to the seizure onset zone. Although they occur a little less frequently, unilateral eye blinking has been reported to lateralize to the ipsilateral side of seizure onset. *Table 5.2* lists the accepted lateralizing symptomatology.

Speech disturbances are also common, either occurring during the seizure or postictally. Vocalizations may be noted during the seizure, comprising of crying, grunting, moaning or humming. Ictal speech is usually clear and understandable and may be repetitive or non-repetitive, usually lateralizing the seizure to the non-dominant hemisphere. Abnormal speech may be characterized by speech arrest during the seizure, in which the patient maintains awareness and experiences dysarthria or dysphasia occurring ictally or postictally. Postictal dysphasia lateralizes to the dominant hemisphere. Patients should always be tested for awareness with vocalization tasks done ictally and postictally, allowing conclusions to be drawn about the presence of speech disturbances.

Head turning has been of questionable lateralizing value with some disputing its reliability. Non-forced head turning occurring at the beginning of a seizure usually lateralizes to the ipsilateral side of the seizure onset; however, these findings have not been proved significant. Forced tonic head turning known as version occurring directly before secondary generalization has been shown to turn reliably to the contralateral side of the seizure onset.

Electroencephalography in temporal lobe epilepsy

The interictal electroencephalography (EEG) characteristically shows abnormal anterior temporal sharp waves, especially in mTLE. In up to 33% of patients, these are bilaterally independent and usually display a characteristic field with a maximum in the basal areas, such as sphenoidal, true temporal or earlobe electrodes.

Ictal onset is usually marked by attenuation of interictal spiking and background; this attenuation can sometimes have lateralizing or even localizing value. Within approximately 30 s of the onset of attenuation, a characteristic 5–7 Hz rhythmic pattern is usually seen in the inferior temporal region. The evolution of this rhythmic synchronized pattern develops usually into intermittent slow waves that ultimately increase in frequency until ictal termination. EEG seizure patterns can display either unilateral or bilateral epileptiform discharges; in the presence of bi-temporal ictal EEG patterns invasive electrodes may identify a unitemporal seizure onset. Auras may always be accompanied by specific EEG changes, although interictal spikes are sometimes noted to disappear.

Specific ictal patterns may help differentiate between mTLE and nTLE. Neocortical temporal seizures are less likely to show clearly localized rhythmical changes in the early stages of the seizure. These seizures also tend to propagate quickly to the ipsilateral mesial structures, explaining the great overlap in clinical manifestations and EEG findings. Sometimes, however, faster or slower frequencies occur in the early stages that can be localized or regionalized.

Neuroimaging

Neuroimaging studies, as with all epilepsy evaluation, plays an integral role in TLE evaluation and diagnosis. The identification of neoplasms, cortical dysplasia, etc. have been previously discussed and present in a similar manner in the temporal lobes as in other areas of the brain. With regard to mTLE, high-resolution, thin-section T1-weighted magnetic resonance imaging can demonstrate hippocampal atrophy in a large number of patients with intractable mTLE. As neuroimaging technology advances, it may be possible to identify architectural changes in the hippocampus causing, for example, sclerosis; in T2-weighted images, hippocampal sclerosis is seen as increased signal.

The use of [18F] fluoro-2-deoxy-D-glucose positron emission tomography (FDG-PET) has proven to be very effective in the identification of temporal lobe foci, especially interictally, with a sensitivity of 84% and a specificity of 86%. Areas of hypoperfusion identify foci, and these areas can be quite large and include more than the epileptogenic zone if the disease is long-standing. Single photon emission computed tomography (SPECT) studies are also used in the identification of epileptogenic foci, although it is usually only used intra-ictally; this is because interictally it is has been demonstrated that it is limited by a low sensitivity. Ictal SPECT may show hyperperfusion in the epileptic focus if the injection is given in the initial phases of the seizure. In mTLE during the immediate postictal phase the mesial structures remain hyperperfused, although the lateral temporal structures are hypoperfused. Within 2–15 minutes postictally there is hypoperfusion throughout the whole temporal lobe and perfusion returns to normal in 10–30 minutes.

Neuropsychological testing in temporal lobe epilepsy

The temporal lobe is associated in general with memory function and, in particular, the hippocampal–diencephalic circuit has been demonstrated to play an important part in declarative memory. The circuit includes the hippocampus and associated mesial temporal structures, the mammillary bodies and the dorsomedial nucleus of the thalamus, and bilateral damage to any of these structures will lead to anterograde amnesia, marked by prominent impairment of explicit memory. Unfortunately those patients who are cognitively most intact before surgery, are those at greatest risk for deficits after surgery. Hence it is important to do extensive neuropsychological testing pre-operatively to ensure accurate advice is given to the patient regarding the risk for memory impairment. Neuropsychological testing should be performed on all patients with epilepsy, not only on those with TLE. It can sometimes provide diagnostic information helping to lateralize or localize the epileptic lesion. Neuropsychological evidence for deficits outside of the proposed seizure onset zone should raise several concerns, as it is associated with poor surgical outcome and should prompt re-evaluation of the proposed hypothesis.

Pre-operative neuropsychological testing provides a baseline assessment of the functioning with which deficits resulting from a long clinical course of epilepsy can be differentiated from the effects of surgery. Minimum testing includes the evaluation of intelligence, frontal executive skills, attention, memory, visuo-spatial skills and language. In left-handed patients an intracarotid amytal test (or Wada test) might be considered in order to assess language lateralization, or those patients whose neuropsychological testing suggests an unusual lateralization. It should be noted, however, that there is a risk of inducing a focal cerebral spasm and infarction in 1 in 200 cases, where available functional magnetic resonance imaging provides a safer alternative.

Aetiology

TLE has a broad range of aetiologies similar to those already discussed in relation to other epilepsies, such as head trauma, neoplasms, brain abscesses and arteriovenous malformations. There are a few, however, who deserve a special mention.

Cavernous haemangiomas are vascular malformations that may occur in isolation or multiply throughout the brain. It is important to note that most patients have a positive family history for these cavernomas and a thorough history may direct the physician at an early diagnostic stage. TLE is not an uncommon sequela to herpes simplex encephalitis, often leading to hippocampal sclerosis and diffuse damage to the temporal lobes. Tuberculoma is one if the most common causes of focal epilepsy in the developing world; however, it is also seen in immunocompromised patients, and such an aetiology should prompt further investigations to rule out HIV infection.

Hippocampal sclerosis has been recognized as the substrate of mTLE. It may be distinguished from other forms of non-specific cell loss through the specific loss of primarily CA1 and hilar neurons, as well as CA2 neurons to a lesser extent. Other characteristic features, such as mossy fibre sprouting and loss of somatostatin and neuropeptide Y containing hilar neurons, help further identify this pathology. Newly sprouted mossy fibres from dentate granule cells aberrantly synapse the dendrites of neighbouring dentate granule cells, creating a recurrent excitatory circuit. Excitation interneurons that normally activate inhibitory interneurons appear to be vulnerable to brain insults. There is a strong association of hippocampal sclerosis with febrile convulsion with up to 66% of patients reporting prolonged febrile convulsions in early childhood. Hippocampal sclerosis is also associated with microdysgenesis and other dysplastic lesions, such as hamartomas and heterotopias; interestingly, there is no significant association with neoplasms. It is still unclear whether seizures are a result of hippocampal sclerosis or vice versa.

Case studies

Case 1

A 31-year-old woman (**CS 1.1**A–J) has had epilepsy for over 10 years. She had viral encephalitis prior to the onset of her seizures and had been successfully controlled with phenytoin until 3 years ago. Her seizures comprised of an initial sensation of fear, losing awareness and observers reported that she looked around at her environment but did not respond or follow commands; after the seizure she had difficulty speaking. These seizures lasted 60–90 seconds and before surgery occurred approximately several times a week. The patient was admitted to the Epilepsy Monitoring Unit (EMU) and underwent presurgical evaluation. Neuroimaging showed mesial temporal sclerosis on the left and concurred with EEG findings. The left mesial structures were resected and she has remained seizure free on levetiracetam. She did report minor difficulty with word finding after surgery but otherwise did not notice any other cognitive decline postoperatively.

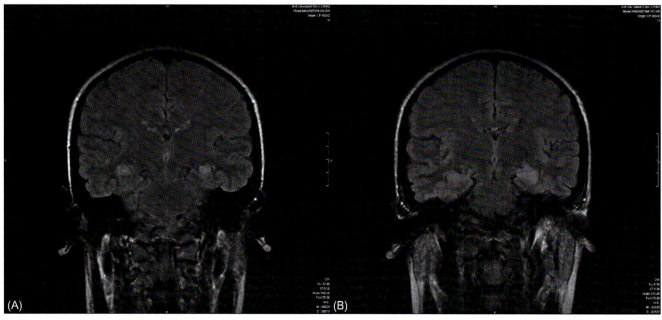

CS 1.1 (A,B) Fluid-attenuated inversion recovery magnetic resonance imaging scans in the coronal plane showing decreased volume of the left mesial structures.

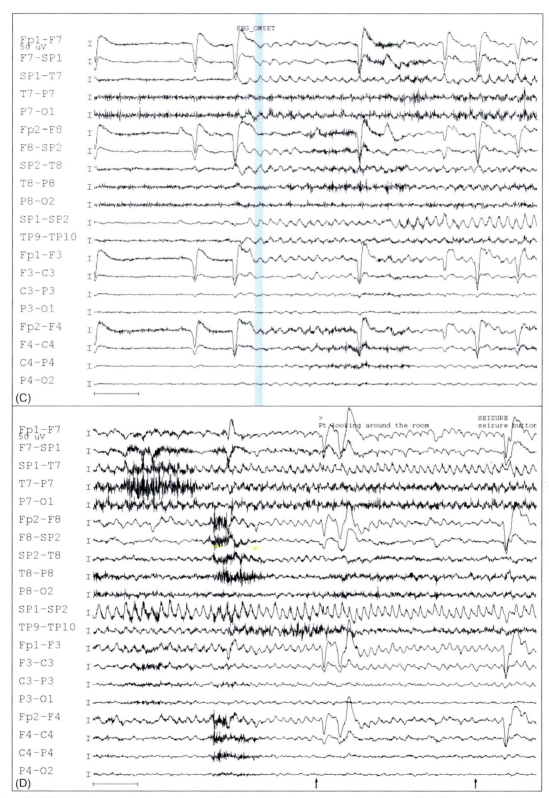

CS 1.1 (*continued*) (C,D) Electroencephalography recording depicting the onset and evolution of a left temporal seizure.

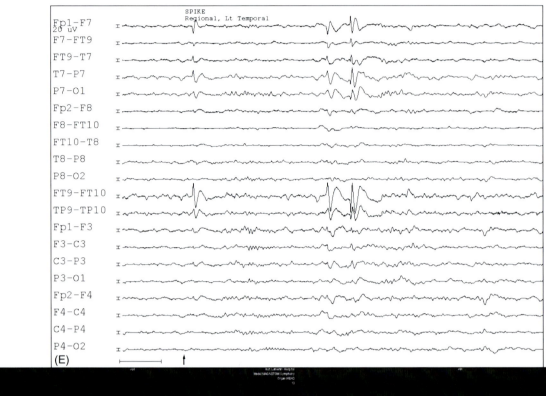

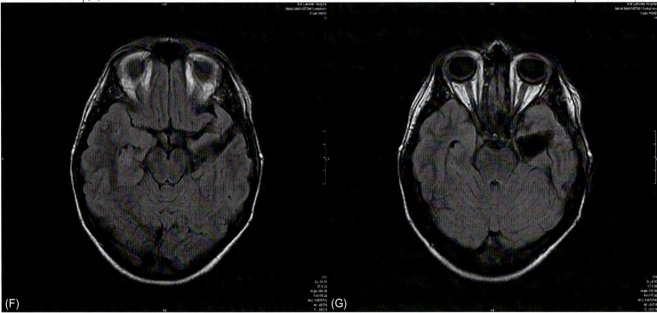

CS 1.1 (*continued*) (E) Electroencephalography recording showing a left temporal spike at FT9. (F–J) T1-weighted magnetic resonance images taken postoperatively showing resection in the saggital, axial and coronal planes.

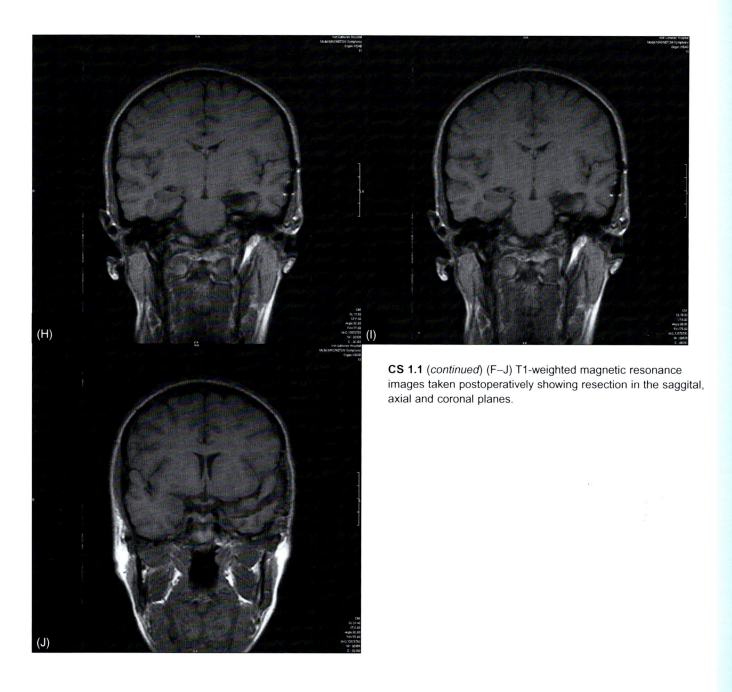

(H)

(I)

(J)

CS 1.1 (*continued*) (F–J) T1-weighted magnetic resonance images taken postoperatively showing resection in the saggital, axial and coronal planes.

Case 2

A 61-year-old woman with epilepsy since she was 1 year old complained of frequent staring spells in which she was unresponsive. These were sometimes preceded by a feeling of numbness and tingling that started in her feet and ascended throughout her body. She suffered generalized seizures only rarely; however, her dialeptic seizures greatly disturbed her everyday life. After failure of a wide range of antiepileptic drugs, pre-surgical evaluation yielded interictal spikes and ictal EEG patterns in the right temporal region (**CS 2.1**A–D) as well as evidence of right mesial temporal sclerosis in the right temporal region (**CS 2.1**E,F). She underwent a right temporal lobectomy and has remained seizure free.

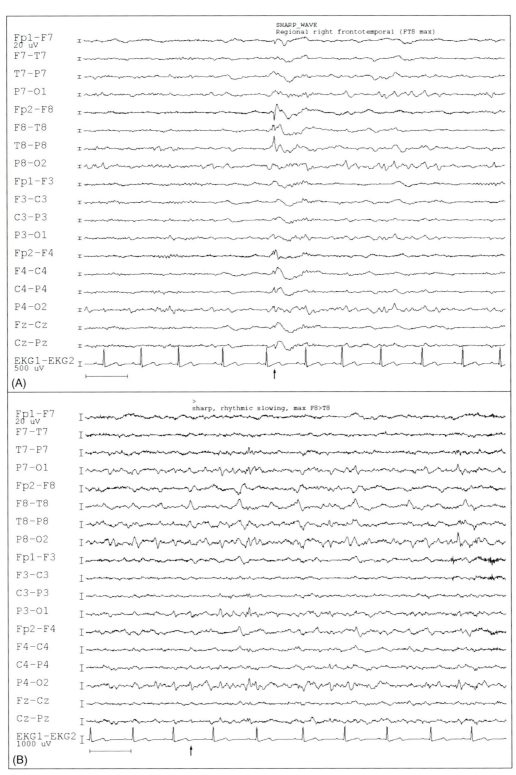

CS 2.1 (A) Depiction of interictal sharp wave in the right temporal region with a maximum at FT8. (B) Electroencephalography recording showing sharp rhythmic slowing in the right temporal region.

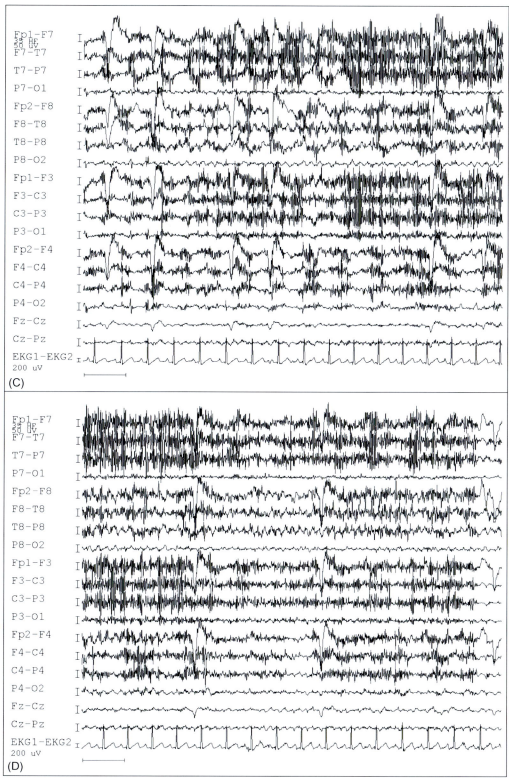

CS 2.1 (*continued*) (C,D) Electroencephalography recording showing seizure pattern localized to the right temporal lobe.

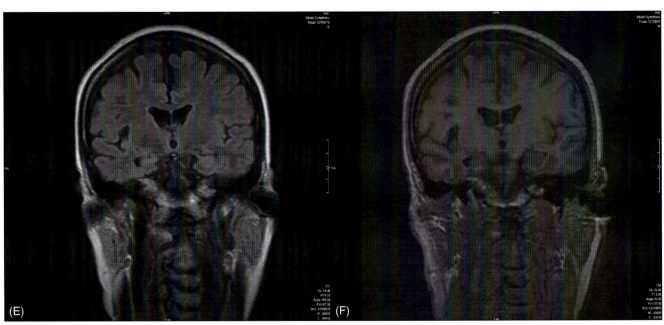

(E)　(F)

CS 2.1 (*continued*) (E) A fluid-attenuated inversion recovery magnetic resonance image in the coronal plane showing decreased volume and signal of the right hippocampus. (F) A T1-weighted magnetic resonance image in the coronal plane showing decreased volume in the right hippocampus.

Case 3 (see opposite)

A 16-year-old female patient presented with episodes of staring and unresponsiveness preceded by a feeling of nausea in her abdomen. Typical risk factors for epilepsy could not be applied to her. Neuroimaging displayed a tumour near the right amygdala and it was promptly excised. The patient remained seizure free for almost 2 years when the auras returned. Upon evaluation, EEG studies showed the ictal patterns to localize to the left temporal lobe; however, neuroimaging showed cystic growth along the boundary of the old resection. The cystic growth was resected, although EEG data contradicted the hypothesis that this was the seizure onset zone and the patient has remained seizure free (**CS 3.1**A–J).

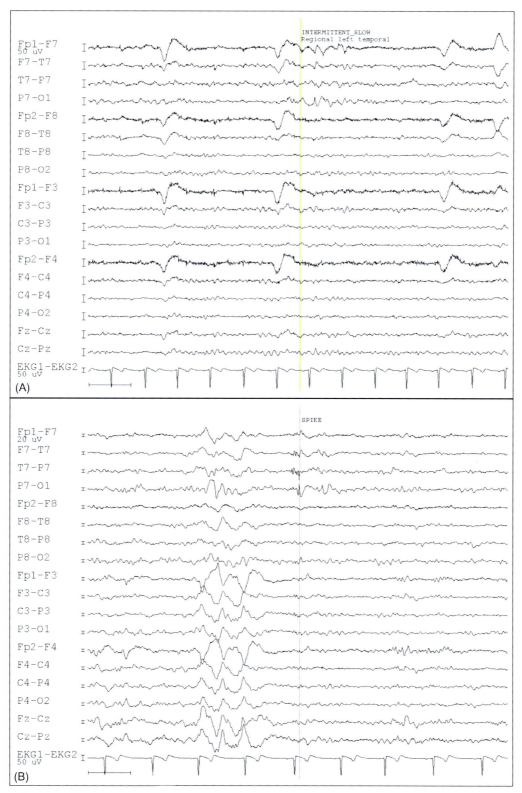

CS 3.1 (A) Displays interictal slowing localized to the left temporal region. (B) Electroencephalography (EEG) recording showing a polyspike with maximum at P7.

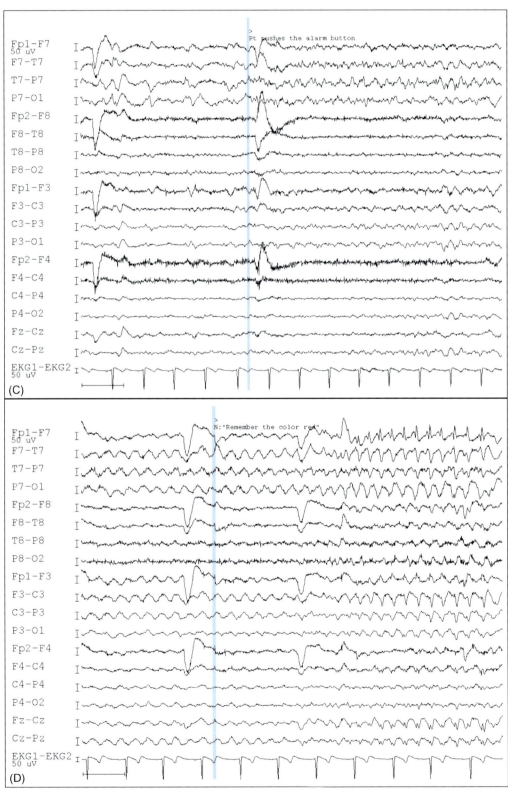

CS 3.1 (*continued*) (C) An EEG depicting onset of a seizure lateralizing to the left. (D) Depicts a different epoch later in the seizure localizing the ictal pattern to the left temporal lobe.

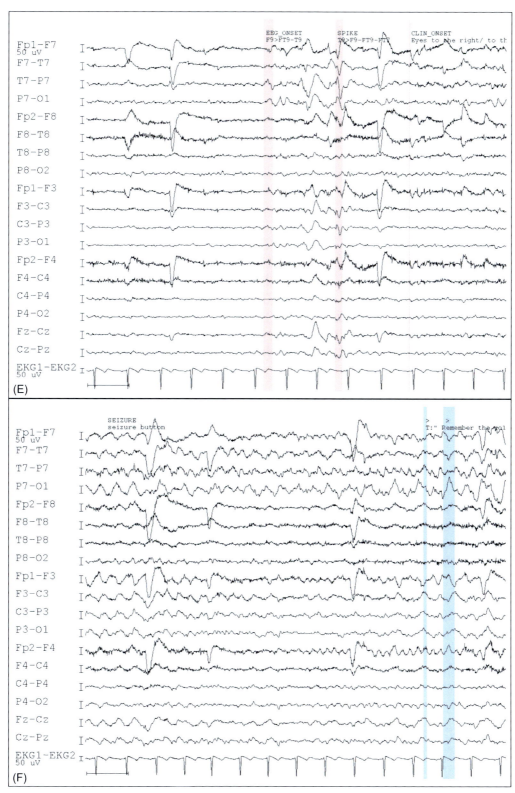

CS 3.1 (*continued*) (E) These show two different epochs in a clinical seizure with the EEG recordings localizing it to the left temporal lobe. (F) These show two different epochs in a clinical seizure with the EEG recordings localizing it to the left temporal lobe.

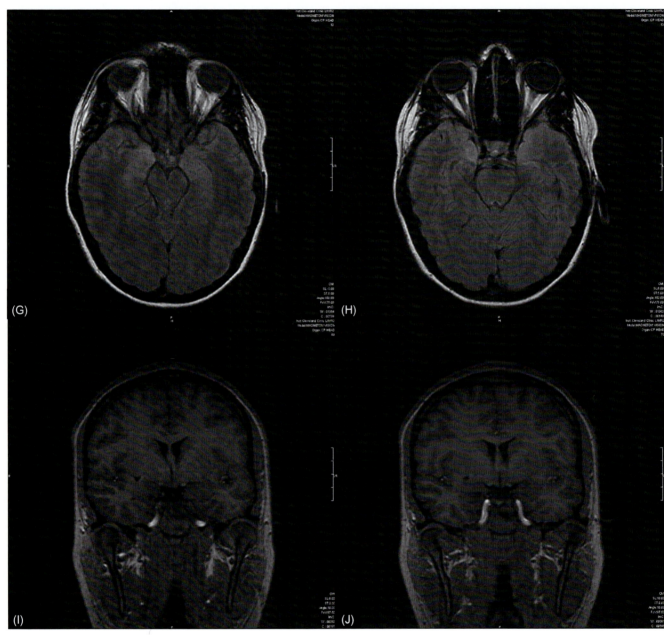

CS 3.1 (*continued*) (G,H) Fluid-attenuated inversion recovery magnetic resonance images in the axial plane showing a tumour near the right amygdala. (I) A T1-weighted image in the coronal plane showing a tumour near the right amygdala. (J) A T1-weighted magnetic resonance image with gadolinium in the coronal plane, which shows no enhancement of the tumour near the right amygdala.

Case 4

A 43-year-old male patient was diagnosed with left TLE 9 years previously. His seizures started with a psychic aura followed by an automotor component and finally by a generalized motor component. He has many risk factors, including head trauma due to recreational boxing, and has a daughter with right TLE. The neuroimaging done at the time failed to show any cortical abnormalities and the patient was deemed not to be suitable for surgery. A vagus nerve stimulator was implanted and found to decrease the seizure frequency by approximately 50%. However, in time it was noticed that the vagus nerve stimulator began to worsen the patient's sleep apnoea and was consequently removed. Upon new evaluation for his epilepsy, neuroimaging showed a slight increase in the signal and volume of the left amygdala with normal hippocampal volume and signal and, once more, no significant temporal or extratemporal abnormalities (**CS 4.1**A). PET scan showed hypometabolism in the left anterior temporal lobe. These findings were confirmed by scalp EEG studies (**CS 4.1**B). The patient then underwent an invasive evaluation with placement of subdural grids covering the left basal temporal, left lateral temporal, left temporal pole, left lateral frontal and left orbitofrontal lobes as well as depth electrodes in the left temporal pole, left amygdala and left hippocampus (**CS 4.1**C–E). The epileptic zone could be identified to the left anterior temporal lobe and a tailored resection was performed. The patient remains seizure free.

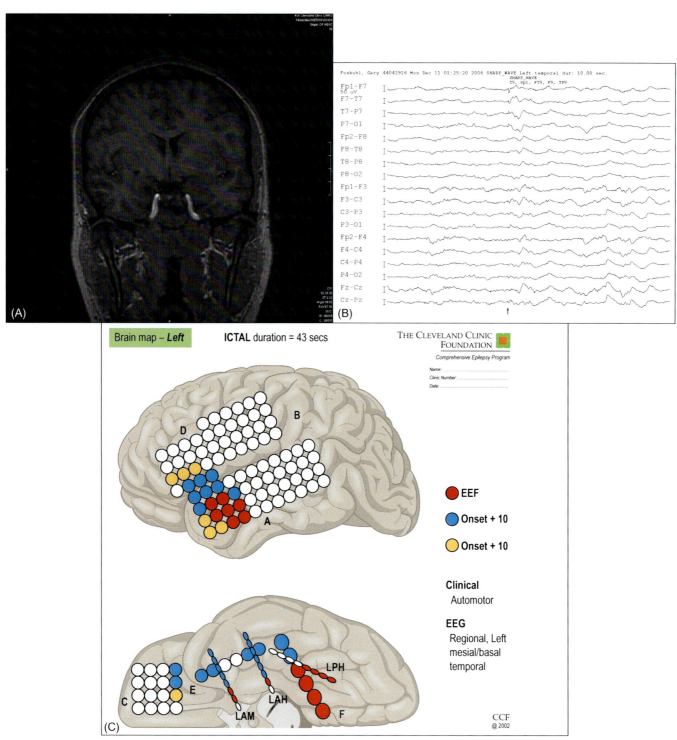

CS 4.1 (A) A T1-weighted magnetic resonance image showing a slight increase in volume of the left hippocampus. (B) A typical scalp electroencephalography recording showing the distribution of a sharp wave through the left temporal chain. (C) Shows the placement of subdural grids and depth electrodes. It also summarizes ictal and interictal electroencephalography findings with respect to electrode placement.

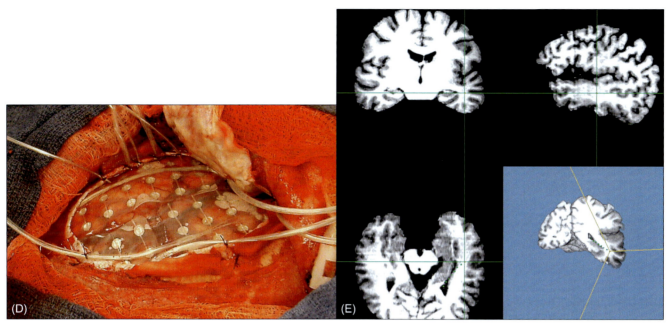

CS 4.1 (*continued*) (D) An intra operative photograph of the subdural grid placement along the lateral extent of the left temporal lobe. (E) A virtual representation of the placement of a depth electrode using stereotaxy and a previous magnetic resonance imaging study.

Conclusions

TLE is the most prevalent epilepsy among adults and may be further classified into mTLE and nTLE. Both syndromes distinguish themselves from other epilepsies through distinctive complex partial seizure semiologies. However, they differ in aetiology, with nTLE arising from a broad range of pathologies and mTLE's pathological substrate being identified as hippocampal sclerosis. Surgical treatment has proven extremely effective in seizure control but poses some challenges to the neurosurgeon. As with all surgeries, careful pre-operative counselling is extremely important in the patient's management, especially with regard to memory deficits and possible visual field cuts subsequent to surgery.

Further reading

Engle J Jr, Pedley TA (eds). *Epilepsy: A Comprehensive Textbook.* Associate ed., Aicardi J. Philadelphia: Lippincott-Raven; 1999.

Kotagal P, Lüders HO (eds). *The Epilepsies: Etiologies and Prevention.* San Diego: Academic Press; 1999.

Lüders HO, Comair Y (eds). *Epilepsy Surgery.* New York: Lippincott, Williams and Wilkins; 2001.

Lüders HO, Noachtar S (eds). *Epileptic Seizures: Pathophysiology and Clinical Semiology.* New York: Saunders; 2000.

Noachtar S, Pfänder M, Arnold S, *et al.* Different seizure patterns in frontal and temporal lobe epilepsy. *Epilepsia* 1998; **39**: 113.

O'Dwyer R, Silva Cunha JP, Vollmar C, *et al.* Lateralizing significance of quantitative analysis of head movements before secondary generalization of seizures of patients with temporal lobe epilepsy. *Epilepsia* 2007; **48**: 524–30.

Pfänder M, Arnold S, Henkel A, *et al.* Clinical features and EEG findings differentiating mesial from neocortical temporal lobe epilepsy. *Epileptic Disord* 2002; **4**: 189–95.

Rosenow F, Lüders HO. Presurgical evaluation of epilepsy. *Brain* 2001; **124**: 1683–700.

Shorvon SD (ed.). *Handbook of Epilepsy Treatment: Forms, Causes and Therapy in Children and Adults,* 2nd edn. Oxford: Wiley-Blackwell; 2005.

Steinhoff BJ, Schindler M, Herrendorf G, Kurth C, Bittermann HJ, Paulus W. The lateralizing value of ictal clinical symptoms in uniregional temporal lobe epilepsy. *European Neurology* 1998; **39**: 72–9.

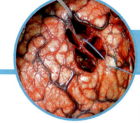

Chapter 6

Insular Lobe Epilepsy

Introduction

Among all forms of epilepsy, insular epilepsy is one of the most rarely reported. Its clinical and electrophysiological characteristics are poorly understood, providing the clinician with many challenges. For a long time, there was great controversy in the literature with some early authors suggesting that seizures arising from the insular cortex could mimic temporal lobe seizures, leading to great confusion between the two seizure types. However, this concept fell out of favour, primarily because the authors in question failed to record spontaneous epileptiform discharges from a focal onset within the insular cortex. In retrospect, the insula's close proximity to the temporal lobe allows, through spread patterns, a considerable overlap in seizure semiology between these two forms of epilepsy. Indeed, many of the difficulties posed arise from the insular lobe's anatomy, especially its

location within the cortex and its prominent connections to other cortical structures. Correct identification and evaluation is extremely difficult and requires astute interpretation of clinical findings; many of the usual tools, such as electroencephalography (EEG) or seizure semiology used by an epileptologist fail to yield exact identifying information.

Anatomy of the insular lobe

Good knowledge of insular lobe anatomy is vital for a better understanding of how the insular lobe and opercular epilepsy manifest clinically (**6.1**). The insula is one of the five cerebral lobes and is located deep within each hemisphere. It is buried in the depths of the lateral sulcus and superficially adjacent to the basal ganglia. It is only exposed when the overlying lips of the lateral sulcus, i.e. the frontal, parietal

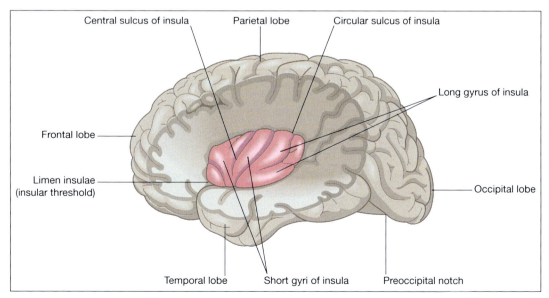

6.1 Lateral aspect of the left insula, exposed by removal of the frontal, parietal and temporal operculum.

and temporal opercula are pulled apart. It is separated from the opercula by a dense wall of arteries running in the lateral fissure. The insula has an approximate triangular surface and is surrounded by the circular sulcus. The ventroanterior margin, the limen insulae, is continuous with the anterior perforated substance in a ventromedial direction.

The insula serves to integrate multimodal information from a broad number of networks. The anterior insula connects with a network of structures that are implicated in oro-alimentary behaviour among other things; connected structures include the piriform cortex, the hippocampus and the amygdala. The posterior insula has dense connections with the primary, the secondary somatosensory cortex and the parietal operculum, structures that together make up a somesthetic network. The connections and consequent functions of the insula can also be distinguished by its cytoarchitecture, divided into three fields: (1) agranular field (Ia, related to olfactory and autonomic functions); (2) dysgranular field (Id, related to gustatory functions); and (3) granular field (Ig, associated with somatosensory, auditory, and visual functions). *Table 6.1* summarizes the connections of the insula and its functions.

Seizure semiology

The greatest challenge insular lobe epilepsy poses to the clinician is the similarity of its clinical features to those of temporal lobe epilepsy (TLE). This is not surprising due to its anatomical proximity to the temporal lobe and prominent connections that allow ictal spread to occur within seconds of ictal onset. The semiology is usually highly suggestive of TLE with great overlap; clonic movement and dystonic posturing have been frequently reported. Insular seizures tend to show visceral sensory, somatosensory and visceral motor phenomena, sometimes reminiscent of auras reported in TLE. Automatisms are also prominent in both TLE and insular lobe epilepsy, with lip smacking highly suggestive of propagation to the amygdala in the latter. An important difference is that in a purely insular seizure with no propagation, awareness is maintained throughout unlike a temporal lobe seizure; however, it may be lost if spread occurs early in the seizure evolution. *Table 6.2* groups prominent seizure semiology that should suggest to the clinician an insular ictal onset zone.

The list in *Table 6.2* is by no means complete; however, on review of case reports, these symptoms appear to be the most prominent and useful while guiding clinicians towards diagnoses, especially those regarding the throat, including

Table 6.1 Connectivity and functions of insula	
Connection to:	**Associated function**
Cerebral cortex	Visceral sensory area
orbital cortex	1° cortical gustatory
frontal operculum	area
lateral premotor cortex	sensations
ventral granular cortex	involving, e.g. throat,
medial area 6	oesophagus
2nd somatosensory	Somatosensory area
area	Visceral motor area
temporal pole	role in vomiting
superior temporal	cardiovascular function
sulcus	Ocular movements area
parietal lobe	
Limbic area	Limbic integrating cortex
cingulate cortex	ongoing behaviour
perirhinal cortex	emotion
entorhinal cortex	
periamygdaloid cortex	
anterior hippocampus	
Amygdaloid nuclei	
lateral	
lateral basal	
central	
cortical	
medial	
Basal ganglia	Vestibular and pain area
dorsal thalamus	
striatum	
Hypothalamus	

excessive salivation. Later stages of the seizure might mimic a temporal lobe seizure with prominent motor phenomena, indicative of ictal spread.

Electroencephalography in insular lobe epilepsy

Again, due to the anatomical situation of the insular lobe surface EEG findings are misleading, often suggesting an ictal onset zone in the temporal lobe. Surface electrodes fail to show specific changes, usually yielding only temporal or

Table 6.2 Insular seizure semiology

Viscerosensitive
  Laryngeal discomfort
  Feeling of strangulation
  Nausea
  Epigastric sensation

Visceromotor
  Lipsmacking
  Chewing

Somesthetic (most often seen on contralateral side)
  Paraesthesiae in face, upper limb, lower limb

Gustatory
  'Bad' taste
  Acid taste
  Salty taste

Speech disturbances
  Dysphonia
  Dysarthria
  Eventual progression to muteness

frontotemporal slowing. To obtain adequate sampling from the insula, depth or subdural electrodes must be used, or intraoperative electrocorticography (ECoG) must be applied. The placement of depth electrodes is not without risk. Depth electrodes must travel through the Sylvian fissure, which contains branches of the middle cerebral artery; to avoid unnecessary complications, usually three-dimensional angiography and magnetic resonance imaging (MRI) (known as stereo-EEG) or computed tomography (CT) integration is carried out to guide their placement. Subdural electrodes are easier to place via the splitting of the Sylvian fissure; however, when placed and confined in this narrow space, often a mass effect from the electrodes themselves is seen and recordings are rendered suboptimal. Placement of subdural electrodes along the mesial temporal lobe structures are also unlikely to record epileptiform discharges from the insula. ECoG is felt by many to be the easiest way to reliably record from the insula. It is performed intraoperatively after the Sylvian fissure has been split; electrodes are placed directly on the insular cortex where a focus can be identified. There are some spatial and time limitations; however, this method has shown itself to yield good electrophysiological data reliably and confirm the clinical suspicion of insular lobe epilepsy (**6.2**).

Some tertiary centres have the capabilities to perform magnetic encephalography, which has been shown to have greater power in identifying deeper foci than surface EEG. Where available and insular epilepsy is suspected, magnetic encephalography might prove to be a useful diagnostic tool.

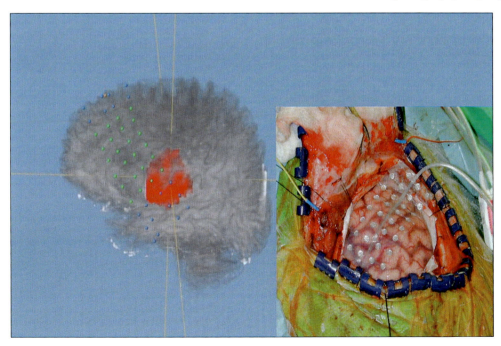

6.2 A three-dimensional reconstruction (left) from magnetic resonance imaging pre-subdural and post-subdural electrode placement with the presence of an insular tumour highlighted in red. Photo (right) taken intraoperatively showing the placement of the subdural electrode grid.

Neuroimaging and aetiology

As with all epilepsies, insular lobe epilepsy has a broad spectrum of aetiologies that with ever improving neuroimaging techniques are being identified more easily. An infectious aetiology is extremely rare and usually a lesional aetiology is sought after. Some aetiologies are accompanied by morbidities that identify them or a syndrome and need only to be confirmed with imaging, e.g. middle cerebral artery haemorrhage. Others are, however, more elusive and require extensive neuroimaging. Low-grade gliomas have been reported several times; it is important to note that regular CT scans usually fail to identify smaller gliomas as well as smaller cavernomas, and MRI, as described earlier in Chapter 1, is required. Cases of cortical dysplasia have also been reported and can be increasingly identified with the use of high-resolution T1-weighted images and fluid-attenuated inversion recovery imaging. An important differentiation between insular lobe epilepsy and TLE is that hippocampal volume loss in the former is rarely appreciated on MRI.

The use of [18F] fluoro-2-deoxy-D-glucose positron emission tomography has also been used successfully to identify insular ictal onset zones. The results from single photon emission CT studies must be considered with great care due to extremely quick spread patterns. If the injection is not performed within the first few seconds of ictal onset, the findings obtained might reflect a spread pattern (often in the temporal lobe) and not an onset zone, possibly resulting in false diagnosis.

Case studies

Case 1

This patient had her first seizure at 27 years of age. She remembered a very prominent sensation of heartburn on falling asleep after which she remembered nothing else. Her husband described her entire body shaking with tongue biting for approximately 1 minute with no loss of urine or bowel control. Her history was insignificant for any risk factors for epilepsy, and other comorbidities included depression and migraine. After failed medical treatment with a number of antiepileptic drugs, she underwent video-EEG monitoring. The evaluation showed seizures that usually started with a long period of coughing and a feeling of nausea; her consciousness then became impaired accompanied by oral automatisms and eye blinking. She then had a head version to the right, followed by tonic posturing of the entire body before a brief clonic phase and final generalized tonic–clonic phase.

Surface EEG located the seizure onset to the left anterior temporal lobe (**CS 1.1**A–G). There were no signal abnormalities seen with MRI-fluid-attenuated inversion recovery imaging, and positron emission tomography scans showed hypometabolism of the left temporal lobe. Invasive evaluation with depth electrodes and subdural grids followed (**CS 1.1**H–J), locating the onset to the superior temporal sulcus and middle temporal gyrus in some seizures and to the left hippocampus in others. Owing to the inconsistent seizure onset and the consistent prominent coughing during her

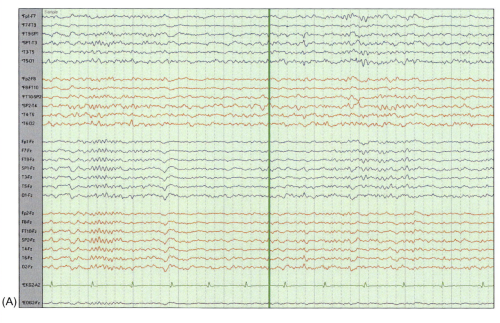

(A)

CS 1.1 (A) Electroencephalography (EEG) recording in a bipolar longitudinal montage showing an interictal left temporal spike.

seizures some members of the team felt that these seizures could have had an insular onset, which would explain the incongruent ictal onsets and seizure semiology. Recording was thus continued. After the recording of more seizures, it was agreed that the seizure onset was insular. The patient was given the following options: (1) removal of electrodes without resection; (2) standard left temporal lobectomy, including mesial structures, acknowledging a high risk of memory decline; or (3) small neocortical resection around the left middle gyrus, acknowledging that the entire epileptogenic zone would not be removed. The patient chose the third option and it was accordingly resected. She has remained seizure free since the resection and is neurologically intact.

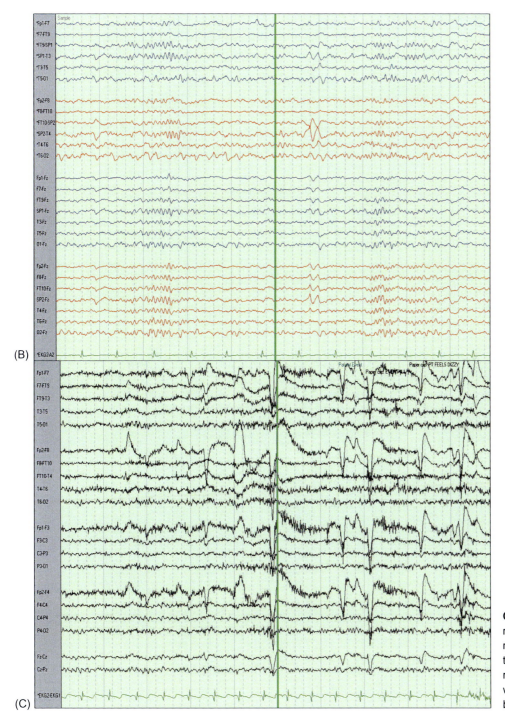

CS 1.1 (*continued*) (B) An EEG recording in a bipolar longitudinal montage showing an interictal right temporal spike. (C) A scalp EEG recording marked by a green line when the patient pressed the seizure button.

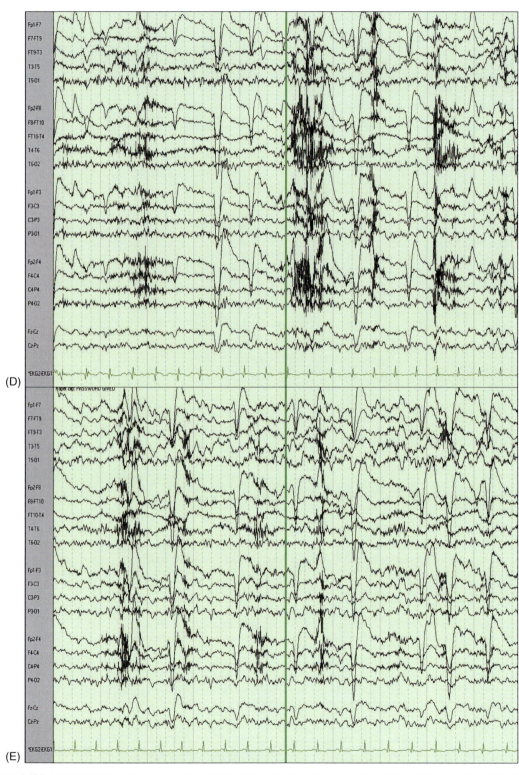

(D)

(E)

CS 1.1 (*continued*) (D) Approximately 10 seconds later theta activity is seen to develop at T3, which spreads within 5 seconds to involve the left temporal chain, as seen in (E–G), the seizure lasting a total of 37 seconds.

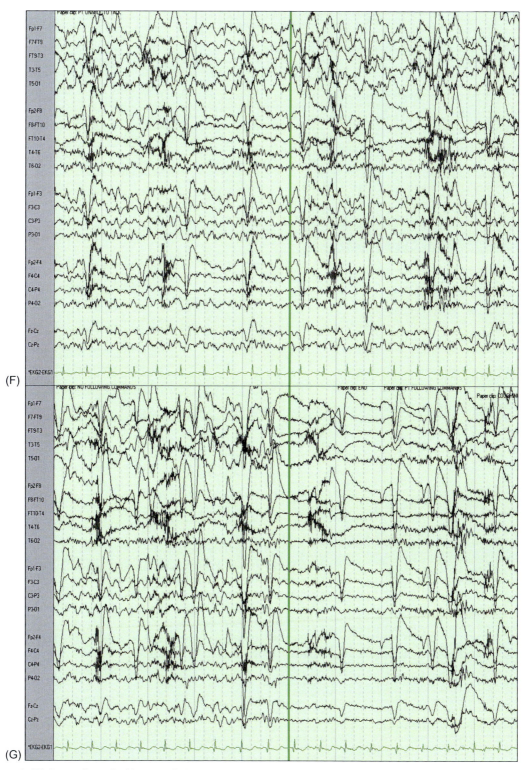

(F)

(G)

CS 1.1 (*continued*) (D) Approximately 10 seconds later theta activity is seen to develop at T3, which spreads within 5 seconds to involve the left temporal chain, as seen in (E–G), the seizure lasting a total of 37 seconds.

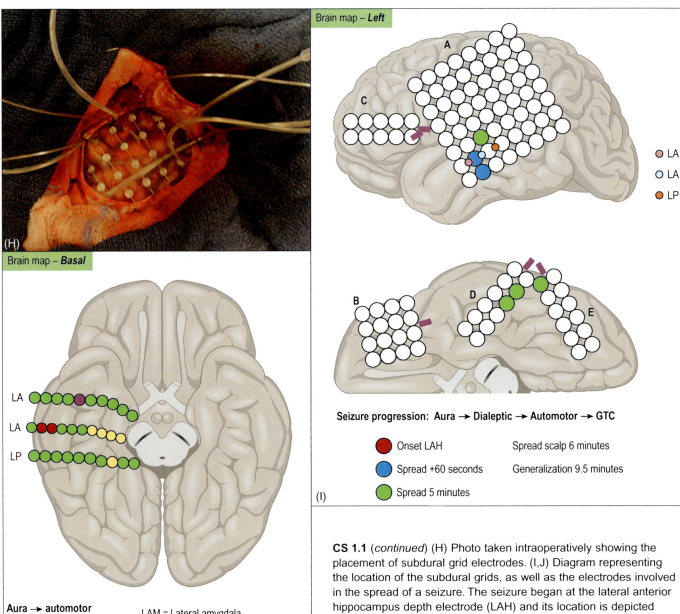

(H)

Brain map – *Left*

A

C

○ LA
○ LA
○ LP

Brain map – *Basal*

LA
LA
LP

B   D   E

Seizure progression: Aura → Dialeptic → Automotor → GTC

● Onset LAH   Spread scalp 6 minutes

● Spread +60 seconds   Generalization 9.5 minutes

● Spread 5 minutes

(I)

Aura → automotor

● Onset LAH

LAM = Lateral amygdala
LPH = Lateral posterior hippocampus

(J)

CS 1.1 (*continued*) (H) Photo taken intraoperatively showing the placement of subdural grid electrodes. (I,J) Diagram representing the location of the subdural grids, as well as the electrodes involved in the spread of a seizure. The seizure began at the lateral anterior hippocampus depth electrode (LAH) and its location is depicted in (J) along with the other depth electrodes. LAH, lateral anterior hippocampus; LAM, lateral amygdala; LPH, lateral posterior hippocampus.

Case 2

The patient's seizures began at age 24 years and proved to be pharmacoresistant to several antiepileptic drugs. His main seizure type at the time of presentation comprised a left chest and arm somatosensory aura, described as a feeling of emptiness that is then followed by tonic posturing of the left arm and then secondarily generalized. Scalp EEG monitoring showed the seizure onset zone to be difficult to localize exactly, localizing it broadly to the right temporal region. MRI failed to show any abnormalities. Ictal single photon emission CT correlated with the EEG showing areas of hyperperfusion in the bilateral anterior frontal and posterior temporal regions, as well as correlating to the positron emission tomography scan, which showed hypometabolism of the posterior right temporal region. Invasive evaluation was performed with placement of a depth electrode in the right insular area and right posterior cingulate region, as well as subdural electrode placement over the right temporal and frontal regions (**CS 2.1**A–D). The epileptogenic zone was located to the right insular cortex. Resective surgery (**CS 2.1**E) was performed

after detailed functional mapping and the patient has remained seizure free since then.

Conclusions

Insular lobe epilepsy is one of the most difficult epilepsies to correctly identify clinically and requires complex electrophysiological invasive recordings to be proven. Failure to identify it might explain why some patients have failed temporal lobectomy. In the setting of what appears to be TLE, some semiologies might suggest insular involvement. Where the insula is suspected, further invasive investigation, usually in the form of ECoG must be performed as it offers patients with insular lobe epilepsy the opportunity to be resected without the risk of all deficits that might ensue after a temporal lobectomy. Clearly, we know very little about the insular lobe in comparison with other lobes and there is much scope for further research, especially in the realm of this most elusive epileptic syndrome.

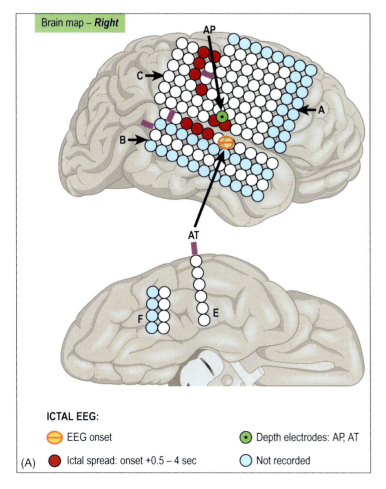

Brain map – *Right*

AP

C

A

B

AT

F   E

ICTAL EEG:

⊖ EEG onset

● Ictal spread: onset +0.5 – 4 sec

◉ Depth electrodes: AP, AT

○ Not recorded

(A)

CS 2.1 (A) Diagram representing the placement of subdural electrodes arranged on plates A–E, as well as the surface location of two depth electrodes named AP and AT. This also shows the electroencephalography (EEG) onset of a seizure as recorded by the subdural electrodes and its spread pattern.

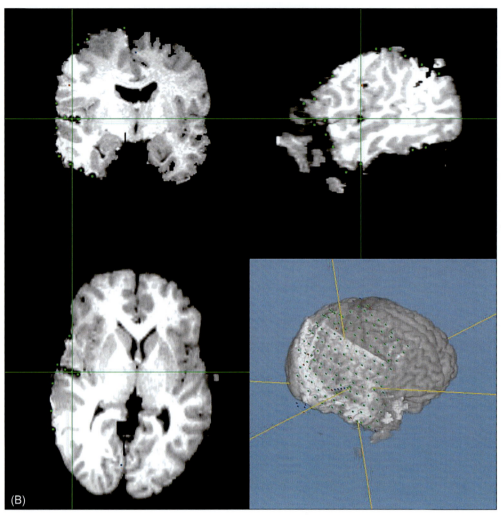

(B)

CS 2.1 (*continued*) (B) A reconstruction using a previous magnetic resonance image of the brain and recording of the electrodes with reference to certain anatomical points shows the placement of the right insula depth electrode named RAT.

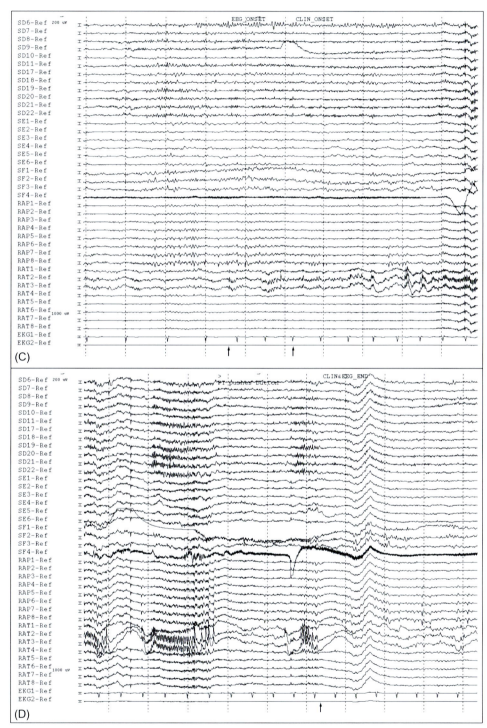

CS 2.1 (*continued*) (C,D) 20 seconds of EEG recording from subdural grids D, E and F, and depth electrodes AP and AT, showing the EEG onset of the seizure starting at electrode AT5 in the right insula and its subsequent spread.

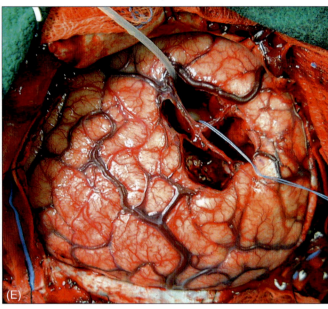

(E)

CS 2.1 (*continued*) (E) A photo taken intraoperatively that shows the completed resection.

Further reading

Guenot M, Isnard J, Sindou M. Surgical anatomy of the insula. *Adv Tech Stand Neurosurg* 2004; **29**: 265–88.

Isnard J, Guenot M, Ostrowsky K, Sindou M, Mauguiere F. The role of the insular cortex in temporal lobe epilepsy. *Ann Neurol* 2000; **48**: 614–23.

Isnard J, Guenot M, Sindou M, Mauguiere F. Clinical manifestations of insular lobe seizures: a stereo-electroencephalographic study. *Epilepsia* 2004; **45**: 1079–90.

Kaido T, Otsuki T, Nakama H, *et al.* Complex behavioral automatism arising from insular cortex. *Epilepsy Behav* 2006; **8**: 315–19.

Ostrowsky K, Isnard J, Ryvlin P, Guenot M, Fischer C, Mauguiere F. Functional mapping of the insular cortex: clinical implication in temporal lobe epilepsy. *Epilepsia* 2000; **41**: 681–6.

Ostrowsky K, Magnin M, Ryvlin P, Isnard J, Guenot M, Mauguiere F. Representation of pain and somatic sensation in the human insula: a study of responses to direct electrical cortical stimulation. *Cereb Cortex* 2002; **12**: 376–85.

Roper SN, Levesque MF, Sutherling WW, Engel J, Jr. Surgical treatment of partial epilepsy arising from the insular cortex. Report of two cases. *J Neurosurg* 1993; **79**: 266–9.

Chapter 7

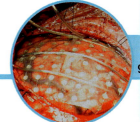

Parieto-Occipital Lobe Epilepsy

Introduction

Epilepsy arising from the posterior cortex poses many challenges to the clinician. Occipital lobe and parietal lobe epilepsies are defined as epilepsy whose ictal discharges arise from the occipital and parietal lobes respectively. These epilepsy syndromes are rare; one study showed a prevalence of 8% for occipital lobe epilepsy and no more than 5% in another study for parietal lobe epilepsy.

A particular challenge in these epilepsies is that many forms of parietal and, occasionally, occipital lobe epilepsy are that the seizure may have very few semiological features that indicate onset in these regions. The clinical semiology of these epilepsies may only manifest following spread to adjacent regions of the cortex. The next challenge arises from usually poorly localizable electroencephalography (EEG) patterns, both interictally and ictally. Again, the EEG findings can arise from the ictal spread, rather than from the ictal onset. A carefully taken history is essential for the correct diagnosis of these epilepsies, as they can easily be misdiagnosed for temporal lobe or frontal lobe epilepsy as well as migraine headaches.

Particular attention should be paid to the symptoms, especially sensory symptoms and auras that occur at the very beginning of seizures, as they usually reveal the useful clinical clues to the localization of the actual ictal onset zone. Unlike most epilepsies the neurological examination can yield important findings that result from the epileptogenic zone. Patients often present with a variety of visual field deficits contralateral to the epileptogenic zone and sometimes are unaware of these deficits. Advances in neuroimaging have also greatly helped to identify possible surgical candidates, which before were either simply diagnosed with cryptogenic epilepsy or misdiagnosed with temporal or frontal lobe epilepsy.

Anatomy of posterior cortex

Parietal lobe

The parietal lobes account for 25% of the brain's volume and only represents 5% of focal epilepsies. The anterior border of the parietal lobe is created by the central sulcus; however, the occipital and temporal borders are more complicated to define. A hypothetical vertical line that cuts the convex surface of both lobes by joining the parieto-occipital sulcus to a shallow depression on the inferior lateral hemispheric border approximately 4 cm from the occipital pole defines the occipital border. An arbitrary line extending posteriorly from the Sylvian fissure to the occipital-parietal line defines the temporal border. See **7.1**.

Occipital lobe

The occipital lobe is the most posterior part of the brain and only occupies approximately 10% of its volume. The arbitrary line that separates the parietal and temporal lobes is continued transversely across the inferior surface of the brain to the parieto-occipital fissure. This lobe is further divided on the medial surface by the calcarine sulcus into the superior lying cuneus and the inferior lying lingual gyrus (**7.1A,B**).

Functional anatomy of the posterior cortex

Parietal lobe

It should be noted that the anatomical definition of the parietal lobe is arbitrary and does not reflect the functionality of the involved cortex. The parieto-occipito-temporal association cortex deals with higher perceptual function

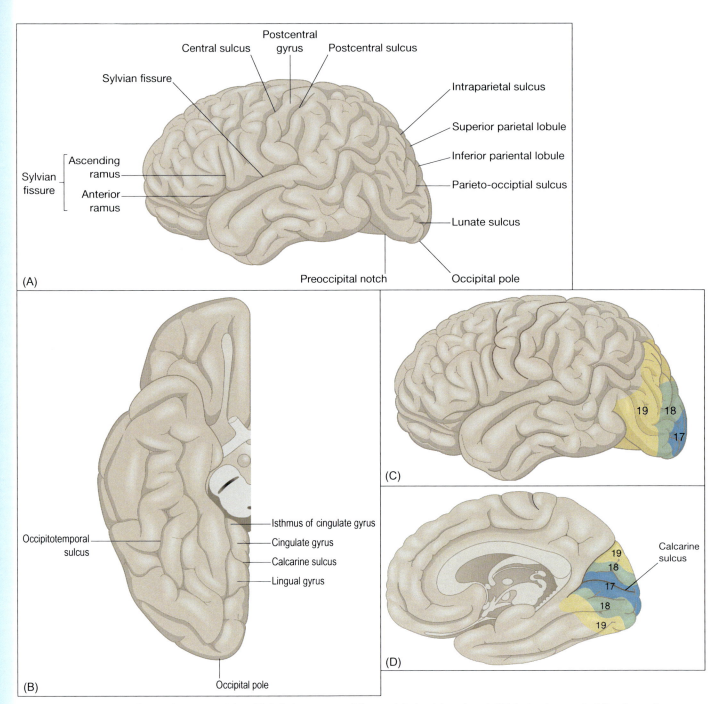

7.1 (A) Lateral aspect of the left occipital lobe. (B) Inferior aspect of the occipital sulci and gyri. (C) Lateral aspect of Brodmann's cortical areas from the left occipital lobe. Area 17 represents the primary visual cortex and areas 18 and 19 represent the visual association areas. (D) Medial aspect of Brodmann's cortical areas of the right occipital lobe. Area 17 represents the primary visual cortex and areas 18 and 19 represent the visual association areas.

and is responsible for the integration of primary sensory inputs to these lobes. The postcentral gyrus runs parallel to the precentral gyrus and represents the somatosensory area. Brodmann divided this gyrus into areas 1, 2, 3a and 3b, which are all important in different aspects of somatic sensation. Topographical representation of contralateral body parts is found here, supramedially for the foot and leg and for the arm, hand and face as one moves in the lateral direction. A second somatosensory area with mainly contralateral (although bilateral representation is minimally present) somatotropic representation is found on the superior border of the Sylvian fissure. This area also serves taste and is located adjacent to the sensory cortex for the tongue and pharynx. The third somatosensory area is located in the posterior parietal lobe; it relates sensory and motor information and integrates the different somatic sensory modalities for perception (7.1). Lesions in the left angular gyrus can lead to Gerstmann's syndrome, which is a tetrad of finger agnosia, right–left confusion, agraphia and acalculia.

Occipital lobe

The cortex of this lobe represents most modalities of vision; it is responsible for the perception of colours and movement as well as other complex aspects of vision, including the association of present and past visual experiences. The primary visual cortex borders inferiorly the calcarine sulcus, topographically representing the visual fields. Brodmann's area 17 corresponds to the primary visual cortex and the visual association cortices are formed by Brodmann's areas 18 and 19 (7.1C).

Seizure semiology

The characteristic phenomena of seizures arising from the parietal and occipital lobes can be subjective sensations, as these lobes primarily subserve sensory perception. Seizure semiology may be divided into positive and negative sensory phenomena, with patients reporting sensations when none are occurring or the feeling of the inability to move or absence of a limb. *Tables 7.1* and *7.2* list features of seizures with the lobe of their respective ictal onset zone.

Parietal lobe epilepsy

Somatosensory seizures often involve the contralateral face or limbs with a broad spectrum of sensations being reported, e.g. numbness, tingling, thermal sensations of burning, genital

sensations, or cold, vertigo, panic, disturbances in body image and gustatory phenomena. Psychic auras, epigastric sensations and ictal amaurosis suggest that ictal spread to extraparietal regions has already occurred. Single photon emission computed tomography (SPECT) studies have shown a hyperperfusion

---

Table 7.1 Semiology of parietal lobe seizures

Initial semiology of parietal lobe origin
  Contralateral paraesthesias
  Contralateral pain
  Gustatory hallucinations (parietal operculum)
  Loss of tone
  Other less common symptoms
    limb movement sensations, thermal sensations, ideomotor apraxia, sexual sensations
  Non-specific symptoms
    choking, vertigo, nausea, disorientation, language disturbances

Semiology suggesting ictal spread
  Asymmetric tonic posturing
  Arrest reaction
  Automatisms similar to those in mesial temporal lobe epilepsy

---

Table 7.2 Semiology of occipital lobe seizures

Initial semiology of occipital lobe origin

  Elementary visual hallucinations
  Ictal amaurosis
  Eye movement sensation (without detectable movement)
  Contralateral tonic (sometimes clonic) eye deviation
  Prominent forced blinking or eyelid flutter

Semiology suggesting ictal spread

  Focal sensory activity
  Clonic motor activity
  Asymmetric tonic posturing
  Formed visual hallucinations
  Automatisms similar to those in mesial temporal lobe epilepsy

of the anterior parietal lobe with sensorimotor semiology and with staring and altered awareness show a hyperperfusion of the posterior parietal lobe. Ictal spread to the frontal lobes usually results in asymmetric posturing of the extremities, unilateral clonic activity, contralateral version (tonic turning of either eye with or without head resulting in unnatural posturing), and hyperkinetic activity such as myoclonus. Spread to the temporal lobes leads to altered consciousness and automatisms, which are similar to those seen in mesial temporal lobe epilepsy.

Occipital lobe epilepsy

Visual phenomena play a central role in the semiology of occipital lobe epilepsy, especially at the beginning of the seizure. Sensations of ocular movement without any detectable movement, nystagmus, eye flutter and forced eye blinking are typical of such seizures. Visual symptoms may be positive such as coloured or bright elementary hallucinations or they may be negative such as scotomas, contralateral hemianopias and amaurosis. In approximately 75% of children with occipital lobe epilepsy, altered consciousness and motor signs were seen, and contralateral version was seen most frequently. Important seizure propagation patterns include the infra-Sylvian and the supra-Sylvian paths. The infra-Sylvian pattern, which spreads to the temporal lobe, is the most common and associated with automatisms, typical of temporal lobe epilepsy and loss of awareness. The supra-Sylvian pattern spreads to the mesial frontal regions and results in contralateral asymmetric tonic posturing or myoclonus. Other patterns of ictal propagation include lateral propagation, which results in focal motor or sensory seizures.

Electroencephalography in parieto-occipital epilepsy

Parietal lobe epilepsy

EEG findings of parietal lobe epilepsy are unfortunately often poorly localized or mislocalized. Interictal recordings are often normal especially when seizures are simple partial. They may, however, show intermittent slowing, either generalized or lateralized, in the presence of either an underlying structural lesion or localized to the midtemporal region. The interictal abnormalities are seen in 5–20% of cases of parietal lobe epilepsy and may be localized to frontocentroparietal, postero-temporal, parietal, and parieto-occipital regions. It may be seen bilaterally in about 5% of patients. One-third of these patients, however,

displays secondary ictal bilateral synchrony as a clue to the parietal origin of epileptiform activity. An aura may be marked by widespread suppression without a clear focal onset, occasionally followed by sharp waves over the parietal region, spreading to more anterior or posterior regions. Usually, however, ictal patterns depend on the propagation pathways taken and may erroneously suggest a temporal or mesial frontal ictal onset zone.

Occipital lobe epilepsy

Unfortunately, only 8–18% of patients have interictal epileptiform activity that is restricted to the occipital lobes. Widespread epileptiform activity or maximal activity in the posterior regions can be recorded. In 30–50% of patients, independent bi-temporal, bisynchronous frontal spike–wave complexes or bi-occipital activity can be seen. Ictal recordings are marked by diffuse suppression or rhythmic activity, which is usually generalized. However, it may also be localized to the temporo-occipital region. Indeed most studies have shown that a large proportion of patients' seizure pattern recordings can be localized to the temporo-occipital region; however, significantly fewer of these patients' seizure onsets can be localized to the occipital lobe. It should also be noted that epileptiform activity might be activated through photostimulation.

Neuroimaging

High-quality neuroimaging is imperative as in all cases of focal epilepsy, particularly medically refractory focal epilepsy. Advances in magnetic resonance imaging (MRI), positron emission tomography (PET) and SPECT scans have greatly improved the identification of possible epileptic lesions in parieto-occipital epilepsy. Up to 75% of patients with occipital lobe epilepsy have structural abnormalities that are correctly identified by various neuroimaging techniques. Usually the elucidation of the structural lesion also sheds light on the aetiology of the epilepsy—focal cortical dysplasia may now be identified in T2-weighted MRI scans (as with old lesions due to neonatal anoxia) and occipital calcifications due to coeliac disease may also be seen on computed tomography and MRI scans. PET scans have been recognized to accurately and reliably identify through the hypoperfusion epileptogenic zones. SPECT scans performed as early as possible into the seizure are also useful in uncovering an otherwise hidden ictal onset zone in this region.

Aetiology

There is a large spectrum of aetiologies responsible for parieto-occipital lobe epilepsy, which spawns from a variety of pathologies. A large proportion consists of neoplasms, the most common are gliomas and astrocytomas, followed by meningiomas, oligodendrogliomas, angiomas and metastases. Disorders of neuron migration are also becoming more prominent, probably due to improved neuroimaging techniques, which allow other disorders, such as focal cortical dysplasia, to be identified. Gliosis, cystic lesions, microgyria and other congenital malformations are more common in occipital lobe epilepsy. In older patients, vascular pathologies should always be considered. Cerebral infarction involving the middle cerebral arteries is associated with frontal and parietal lobe damage and consequent epilepsy. The parietal lobe appears to be one of the most susceptible parts of the brain to epileptic seizures after intracerebral haemorrhage. Perinatal insults resulting in hypoxaemia or hypoglycaemia have also been associated with occipital lobe epilepsy later in life. The triad of coeliac disease, intracranial calcifications and epilepsy, known by some as Sturge–Weber–Dimitri syndrome has been established as a variant Sturge–Weber syndrome without naevus flammeus, which includes calcifications predominantly found bilaterally in the posterior cortex. Mitochondrial cytopathies as well as other congenital metabolic disorders have been established as causes of parieto-occipital lobe epilepsy.

Case studies

Case 1

The first case is of a 28-year-old right-handed man who has occipital lobe epilepsy with a history of right occipital meningioma. His first seizure was unwitnessed but he remembers going to the bathroom after a long night drinking with friends and then waking up beside the toilet, he assumed that he had blacked out. Three years later he presented to an ophthalmologist with difficulty focusing, bumping into things as well as other visual spatial difficulties. He also reported at this time 'pressure in his head' when he lay down, some unsteadiness of gait and numbness affecting his left side. An abnormal visual field test and increased intracranial pressure prompted a CT scan, which identified a right occipital meningioma that was resected. Postoperatively, he remained seizure free for 7 months when he started to have generalized motor seizures once more. His second seizure also occurred when sleep deprived. Neuroimaging shows postoperative gliosis, which may be the aetiology of the current seizures (**CS 1.1**A–C).

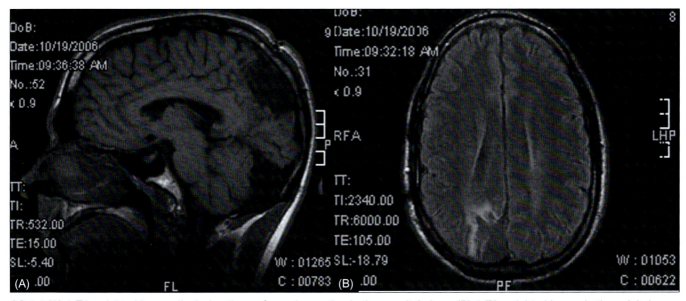

CS 1.1 (A) A T1-weighted image displaying the performed resection in the saggital plane. (B) A T2-weighted image in the axial plane; postoperative gliosis can be seen in the right occipital lobe.

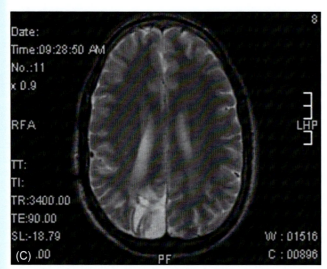

CS 1.1 (*continued*) (C) A postoperative axial view; however, the fluid attenuated inversion recovery method was used, which allows the postoperative gliosis to be easily appreciated.

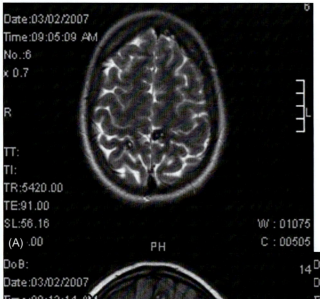

Case 2

This case is a 19-year-old right-handed woman with a 4-month history of somatosensory seizures. She reports that her seizures begin with a warm, 'tingly' sensation on her right knee, which then spreads up the outside of her right arm to the elbow. She then becomes short of breath and light-headed, feeling anxious. She has had one generalized motor seizure, which started as described above, she then became aphasic and although she wanted to, could not call for help. According to a witness, she then became stiff, and all her extremities began to jerk and thrash about, lasting for 14 minutes in total. Postictally she had difficulty walking and was disorientated for a few hours. The above semiology is typical of parietal lobe epilepsy, which was confirmed by neuroimaging when two cavernous angiomas were identified (the largest in the low left medial parietal lobe) (**CS 2.1A–C**). She had a positive family history for cavernous angiomas with her uncle, who also has epilepsy.

CS 2.1 (A) A T2-weighted image showing two cavernous angiomas, the larger being in the left low medial parietal lobe. (B,C) Two adjacent fluid attenuated inversion recovery images in the axial plane showing a large cavernous angioma.

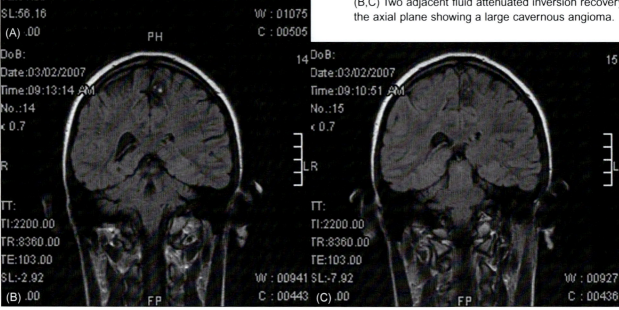

Case 3

This case is a 21-year-old right-handed man whose seizures began at 11 years of age. He has visual auras that consist of a 'blackout' of his vision or if they are minor he is able to see the outline or shadow of objects. These auras may evolve followed by versive eye and head movement to the left; clonic movement of the left arm and then a secondarily generalized tonic–clonic seizure; thus containing many features of occipital lobe semiology. T2-weighted MRI showed increased signal in the right occipital lobe; hypometabolism was seen in this region on the PET scan. Ophthalmological examination found an isolated paracentral scotoma in the right eye and a normal left eye. He was admitted to an epilepsy unit where scalp EEG was first recorded (**CS 3.1**A–D). An invasive evaluation ensued recording from the right occipital, parietal and temporal lobe (**CS 3.1**E,F). This evaluation confirmed the ictal onset zone to be indeed occipital (**CS 3.1**G–L). The patient decided to pursue surgical treatment aware of the risk to his vision. He is now seizure free on phenytoin monotherapy.

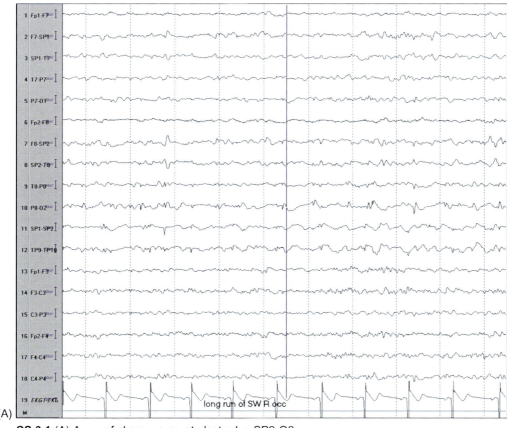

(A)

CS 3.1 (A) A run of sharp waves at electrodes SP2-O2.

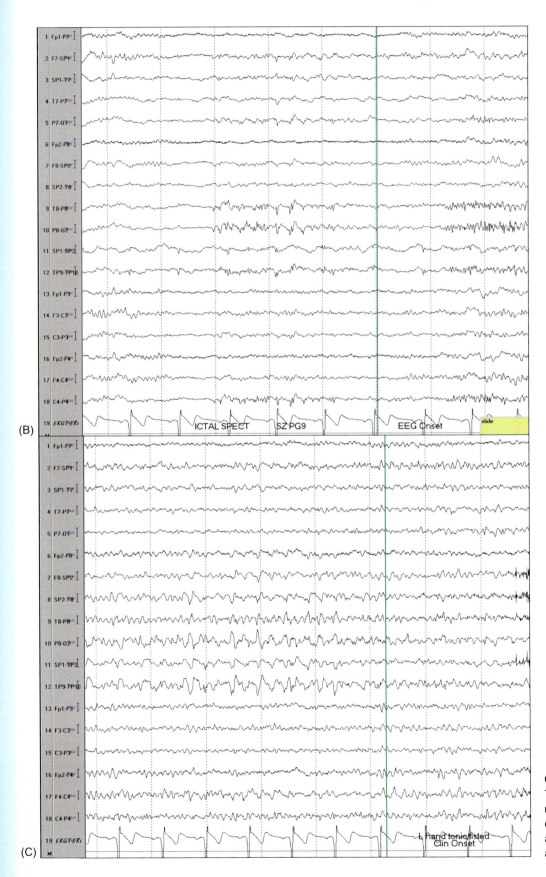

(B)

(C)

CS 3.1 (*continued*) (B–D) The evolution of a seizure measured by scalp electroencephalography (EEG) arising from electrode P8, T8 and O2.

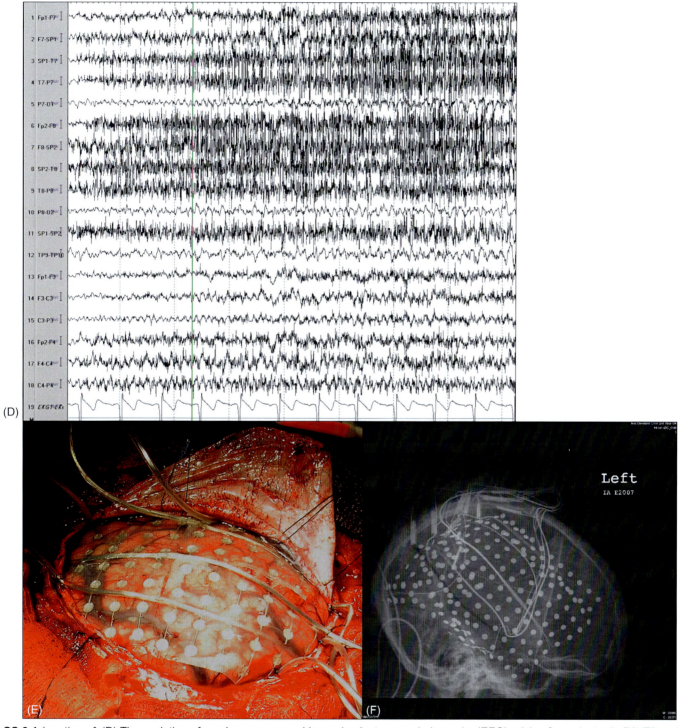

(D)

(E)

(F)

CS 3.1 (*continued*) (D) The evolution of a seizure measured by scalp electroencephalography (EEG) arising from electrode P8, T8 and O2. (E,F) Placement of subdural grids intraoperatively (E) and confirmed by X-ray (F).

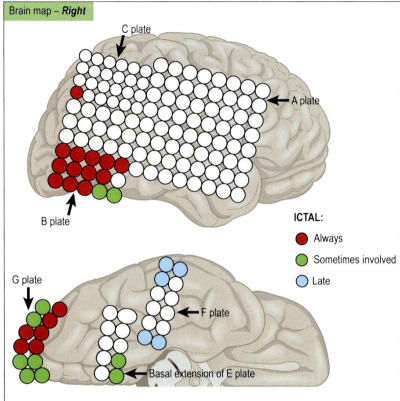

Brain map – *Right*

C plate

A plate

B plate

ICTAL:

● Always

● Sometimes involved

● Late

G plate

F plate

Basal extension of E plate

(G)

CS 3.1 (*continued*) (G) In cartoon form, mapping of ictal onset and spread on subdural grids as defined by ictal EEG findings. (H–L) Evolution of a seizure recorded by subdural grids displayed with a referential montage using scalp reference.

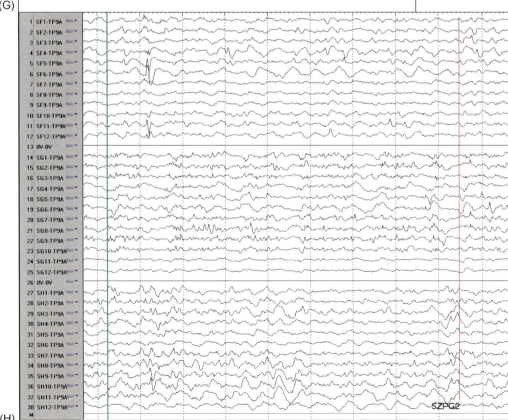

(H)

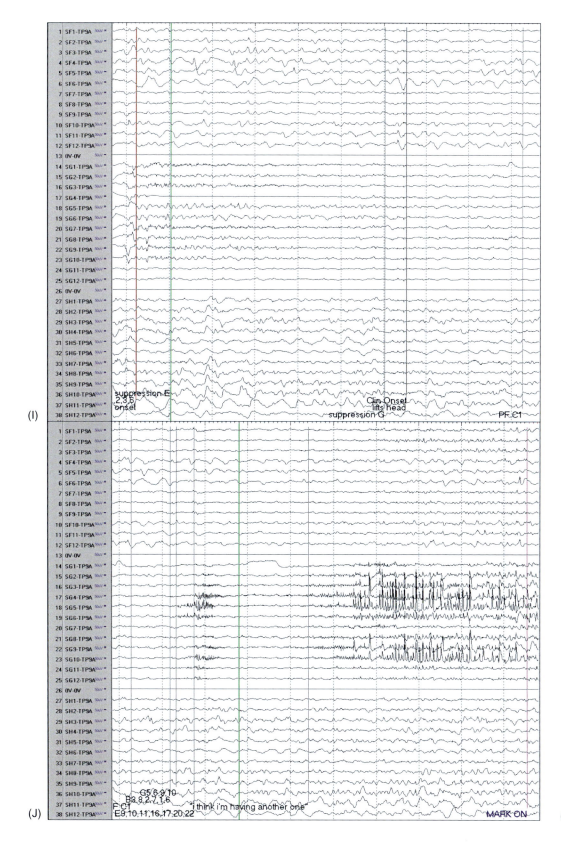

CS 3.1 *(continued)*

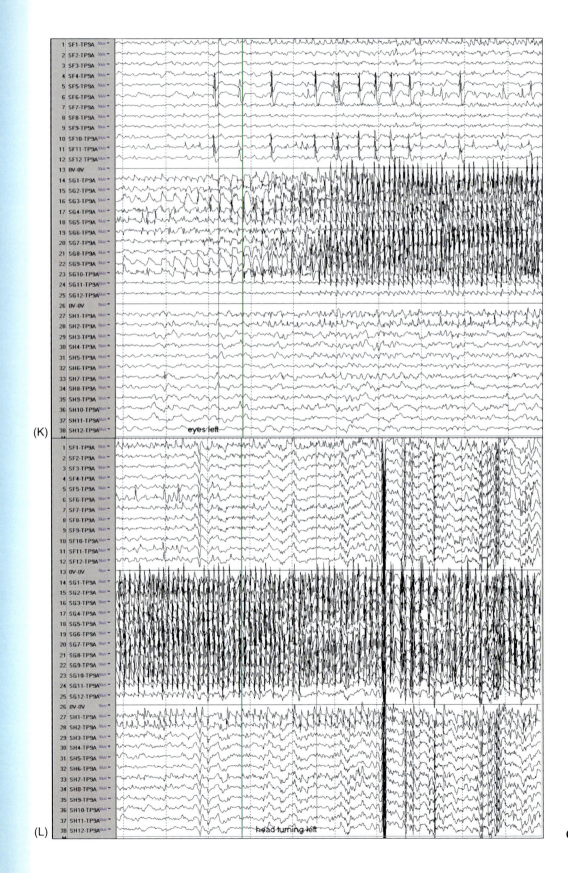

CS 3.1 (*continued*)

Case 4

This case is a 17-month-old boy diagnosed with Sturge–Weber syndrome whose seizures started at 7 months. He met his developmental milestones at the appropriate age for the first 12 months, after which motor developmental delay was noted and at 15 months went into a 45-minute episode of status epilepticus. He was unable to move his left side for 2 weeks after this incident and since then his left arm is in constant flexion; on examination there is persistent left leg weakness and left side neglect. Vision is thought to be impaired after close clinical observation. He displays two seizure types: left clonic movement of the eye, face, and extremities, and dialeptic seizures (**CS 4.1A**). The MRI findings are consistent with Sturge–Weber syndrome; they show asymmetric enhancement of the meninges in the right portion of the posterior cortex and an area of abnormal vascularity in the right parietal region (**CS 4.1B,C**).

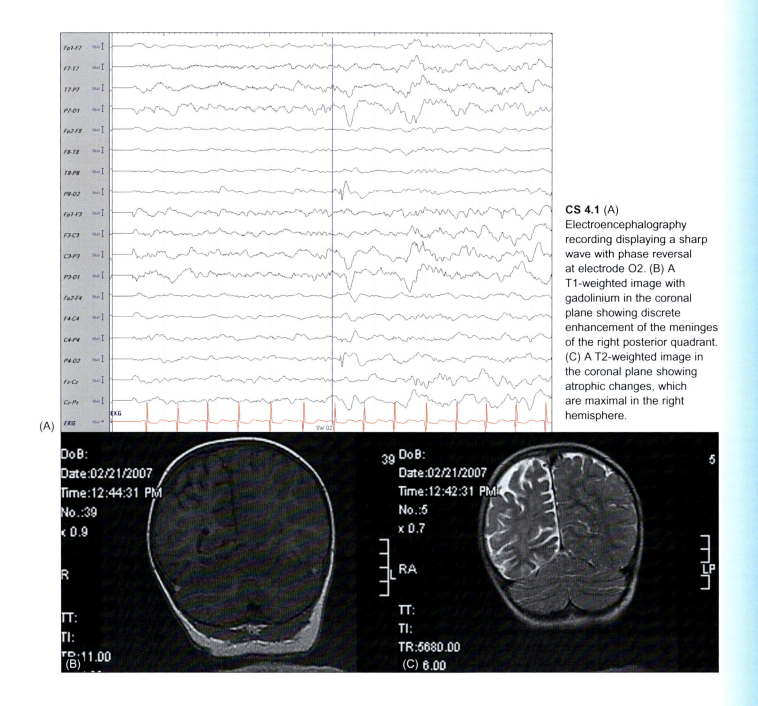

CS 4.1 (A) Electroencephalography recording displaying a sharp wave with phase reversal at electrode O2. (B) A T1-weighted image with gadolinium in the coronal plane showing discrete enhancement of the meninges of the right posterior quadrant. (C) A T2-weighted image in the coronal plane showing atrophic changes, which are maximal in the right hemisphere.

Case 5

This case is a 22-month-old boy who developed seizures at 5 months of age, consisting of spasms with eye blinking, followed by flexion of the trunk, which were accompanied by extension and stiffening of the extremities. The seizures occur in clusters five to six times per day and each cluster lasts approximately 7 minutes (**CS 5.1A–C**). The MRI scan showed loss of normal grey–white differentiation in the right posterior temporal and right occipital lobes and an increased T2 signal in the right parieto-occipital region (**CS 5.1D**). The PET scan confirmed these findings displaying right parieto-occipital hypometabolism involving the inferior parietal lobule extending into the fusiform gyrus (**CS 5.1E**).

Conclusions

Parieto-occipital lobe epilepsy is a rare form of epilepsy presenting several challenges due to poor localization of seizure semiology and EEG findings. Careful history taking and neuroimaging on occasion provides helpful clues to correctly localizing this form of epilepsy. Correct localization can become extremely critical in patients whom medications have failed. There is a group of epilepsies with localization features related to this topic, which were not discussed in this chapter: benign partial epilepsy with centro-temporal spikes, childhood epilepsy with occipital paroxysms, and early onset benign occipital epilepsy (these were discussed earlier in Chapter 1 under 'Aetiology').

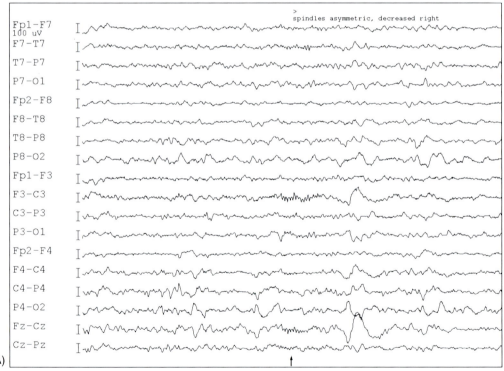

(A)

CS 5.1 (A) Shows an electroencephalography (EEG) sleep recording that demonstrates asymmetric sleep spindles that are decreased throughout the right hemisphere.

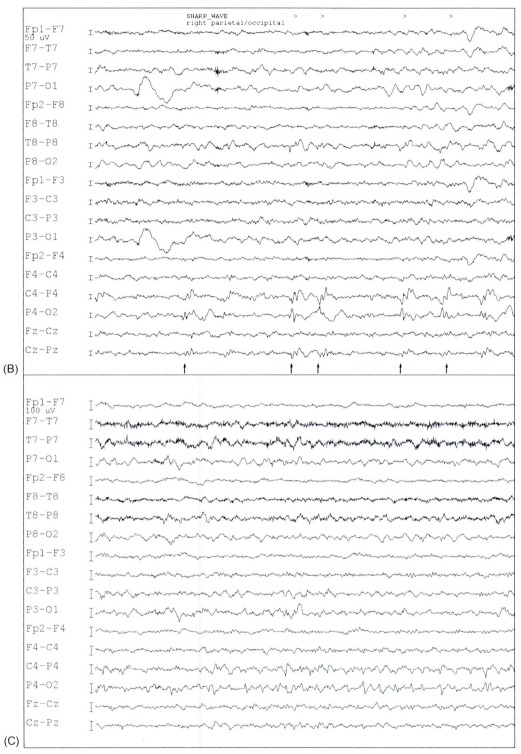

(B)

(C)

CS 5.1 (*continued*) (B) An EEG recording in the awake state displays a run of sharp waves in the right parietal lobe at electrode P4.
(C) Shows another awake EEG recording displaying the onset of a right parietal seizure, arising from electrode P4.

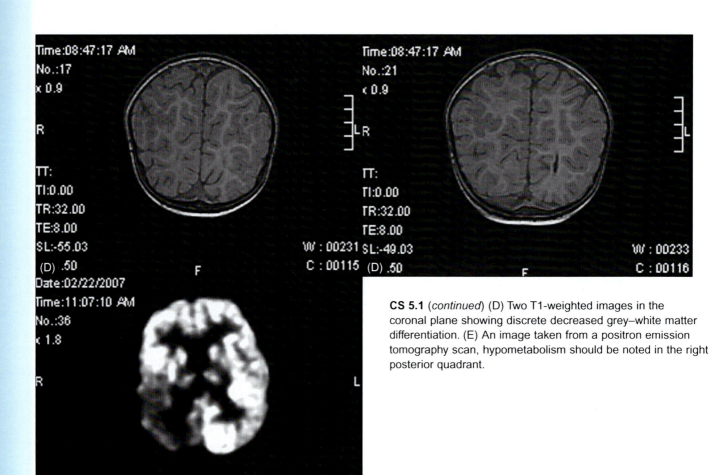

CS 5.1 (*continued*) (D) Two T1-weighted images in the coronal plane showing discrete decreased grey–white matter differentiation. (E) An image taken from a positron emission tomography scan, hypometabolism should be noted in the right posterior quadrant.

Further reading

Acharya JN, Wyllie E, Lüders HO, Kotagal P, Lancman M, Coelho M. Seizure symptomatology in infants with localization-related epilepsy. *Neurology* 1997; **48**: 189–96.

Blume WT, Whiting SE, Girvin JP. Epilepsy surgery in the posterior cortex. *Ann Neurol* 1991; **29**: 638–45.

Boesebeck F, Schulz R, May T, Ebner A. Lateralizing semiology predicts the seizure outcome after epilepsy surgery in the posterior cortex. *Brain* 2002; **125**: 2320–31.

Caraballo RH, Sakr D, Mozzi M, *et al.* Symptomatic occipital lobe epilepsy following neonatal hypoglycemia. *Pediatr Neurol* 2004; **31**: 24–9.

Engle J Jr, Pedley TA (eds). *Epilepsy: A Comprehensive Textbook.* Associate ed., Aicardi J. Philadelphia: Lippincott-Raven; 1999.

Jehi LE, O'Dwyer R, Najm I, Alexopoulos A, Bingaman W. A longitudinal study of surgical outcome and its determinants following posterior cortex epilepsy surgery. *Epilepsia* 2009; **50**: 2040–52. Epub 2009 Mar 23.

Lüders HO, Noachtar S (eds). *Epileptic Seizures: Pathophysiology and Clinical Semiology.* New York: Saunders; 2000.

Nakken KO, Roste GK, Hauglie-Hanssen E. Coeliac disease, unilateral occipital calcifications, and drug-resistant epilepsy: successful lesionectomy. *Acta Neurol Scand* 2005; **111**: 202–4.

Shorvon SD (ed.). *Handbook of Epilepsy Treatment: Forms, Causes and Therapy in Children and Adults*, 2nd edn. Oxford: Wiley-Blackwell; 2005.

Sveinbjornsdottir S, Duncan JS. Parietal and occipital lobe epilepsy: a review. *Epilepsia* 1993; **34**: 493–521.

Werhahn KJ, Arnold S, Mueller A, Ebner A, Winkler PA, Noachtar S. Differences in seizure evolution of tonic seizures in extratemporal epilepsies: possibility to identify different focal syndromes. *J Neurol Sci* 1997; **150**: S97.

Chapter 8

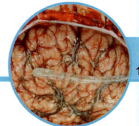

An Overview of Epilepsy Treatment

Introduction

The treatment of epilepsy can be complex, particularly in cases of medically intractable epilepsy. For the purposes of this book, the authors will provide a short and concise synopsis of available treatments for the different broad categories of epilepsy. The medical management of epilepsy starts with a selection of appropriate antiepileptic drugs (AEDs) and if three or more AEDs fail after adequate trials, the epilepsy is termed intractable. At this stage, appropriate surgical options should be considered. A careful review of the treatment history is important to determine if the AED trials were indeed optimal prior to pursuing a surgical option. An AED trial is adequate if control of seizures is achieved with a tolerable dose. An AED trial attempts to address two main issues: seizure control

and tolerability of the medication. This can be achieved by designing titration schedules and determining target doses that should be individualized to each patient.

Table 8.1 lists the most common side effects of regularly used AEDs. Patients most often complain of sedation, double-vision, ataxia and dizziness. Measurement of AED concentrations in plasma can help in guiding medical therapy especially at times of initiation, dose adjustment, appearance of side effects, therapeutic failure, therapeutic success, or with multiple AED usage. However, the clinical effects of some AEDs do not correlate well with their concentrations in the plasma. Recommended concentrations are therefore only to be used as general guidelines for therapy. The clinically relevant AED regimen is then guided by a clinical assessment of efficacy and toxicity.

Table 8.1 Common side effects of AEDs

Drug	Dose related	Idiosyncratic
PHT	Diplopia	Skin rash
	Ataxia	Fever
	Gingival hyperplasia	Lymphoid hyperplasia
	Hirsutism	Hepatic dysfunction
	Coarse facial features	Blood dyscrasia
	Polyneuropathy	Stevens–Johnson syndrome
	Osteomalacia	
	Megaloblastic anaemia	
CBZ	Diplopia	Skin rash
	Ataxia	Hepatic dysfunction
	Gastrointestinal distress	Blood dyscrasia
	Sedation	Stevens–Johnson syndrome
		SIADH
OXB	Hyponatraemia	Skin rash

Table 8.1 Common side effects of AEDs (*continued*)

PHB	Sedation Insomnia Behavioural disturbance Diplopia Ataxia	Skin rash Stevens–Johnson syndrome
VPA	Gastrointestinal distress Tremor Sedation Weight gain Hair loss Thrombocytopenia	Hepatic dysfunction Peripheral oedema
ETX	Gastrointestinal distress Sedation Ataxia Headache	Skin rash Blood dyscrasia
KLN	Sedation Diplopia Ataxia Behavioural disturbance Hypersalivation	
GBP	Drowsiness Fatigue	Drugged sensation Loss of libido
LTG	Dizziness Ataxia	Skin rash (especially with treatment with VPA) Stevens–Johnson syndrome
VGB	Sedation Vertigo Psychosis	Peripheral visual constriction (irreversible)
TPM	Ataxia Confusion	Renal stones Glaucoma
TGB	Dizziness Sedation Nausea	Skin rash
ZNM	Drowsiness Nephrolithiasis	Ataxia Anorexia Headache Skin rash

CBZ, Carbamazepine; ETX, Ethosuximide; GBP, Gabapentin; KLN, Clonazepam; LTG, Lamotrigine; OXB, Oxycarbamazepine; PHB, Phenobarbital; PHT, Phenytoin; SIADH, syndrome of inappropriate antidiuretic hormone secretion; TGB, Tiagabine; TPM, Topiramate; VGB, Vigabatrin; VPA, Valproate; ZNM, Zonisamide.

AEDs are often given concomitantly with other medications, including other AEDs. Drug interactions can occur, some of which are summarized in *Table 8.2*.

Generalized epilepsies

Valproic acid is often effective in patients with juvenile myoclonic epilepsy. It is effective in the treatment of myoclonus and generalized tonic-clonic seizures, as well as absence seizures (ILEA classification). Newer AEDs such as levetiracetam, topiramate or lamotrigine may also be useful. There is some evidence to suggest that myoclonus could be worsened with the use of lamotrigine. Ethosuximide is noted to be effective in controlling absence seizures but does not suppress generalized tonic-clonic seizures. Clonazepam may be helpful in controlling myoclonus but is less effective in controlling generalized tonic-clonic seizures. Carbamazepine, phenytoin, vigabatrin and tiagabine may worsen some seizure types in generalized epilepsy (*Table 8.3*).

The treatment of West syndrome can be challenging and is measured by elimination of spasms as well as hypsarrhythmic EEG patterns. Corticotropin (adrenocorticotrophic hormone) and vigabatrin have been noted to be effective in this disorder. Prompt identification of the syndrome and initiation of treatment may allow for the best possible developmental outcome. However, some patients with infantile spasms have an underlying congenital brain anomaly such as lissencephaly, which precludes normal brain development. Other AEDs such as valproic acid, benzodiazepines, as well as the ketogenic diet and epilepsy surgery can also play a role in therapy. If seizures persist over time, the disease evolves into a Lennox–Gastaut syndrome or some form of focal or multifocal epilepsy. Pyridoxine (vitamin B6) dependence is an infrequent aetiology for infantile spasms. Seizures in these cases are aborted immediately following intravenous administration of vitamin B6.

In cases of Landau–Kleffner syndrome and other encephalopathic generalized epilepsies, treatment is aimed at seizure control, management of associated cognitive or behavioural dysfunction and prevention of physical injuries from seizures. AEDS are often ineffective in the treatment of these epilepsies. Patients are often on multiple AEDs and the occurrence of neurotoxicity is a frequent occurrence. It is helpful to prevent excessive sedation as this often precipitates worsening of seizure frequency. Myoclonus and atonic seizures are typically more easily controlled than tonic

Table 8.2 Interactions of antiepileptic drugs

Drug	Levels increased by:	Levels decreased by:
PHT	Benzodiazepines Chloramphenicol Disulfram Ethanol Isoniazid Phenylbutazone Sulfonamides TPM Trimethoprim Warfarin ZNM	CBZ PHB Pyridoxine VGB
CBZ	Erythromycin Felbamate Isoniazid Propoxyphene VPA	PHB PHT OXB ZNM
PHB	Primidone VPA	
VPA	–	TPM TGB LTG PHT CBZ
ETX	VPA	–
KLN	–	–
GBP	–	–
LTG	VPA	CBZ PHB PHT
VGB	–	–
TPM	–	CBZ PHT PHB
ZNM	LTG	CBZ PHT

CBZ, Carbamazepine; ETX, Ethosuximide; GBP, Gabapentin; KLN, Clonazepam; LTG, Lamotrigine; OXB, Oxycarbamazepine; PHB, Phenobarbital; PHT, Phenytoin; TGB, Tiagabine; TPM, Topiramate; VGB, Vigabatrin; VPA, Valproate; ZNM, Zonisamide.

Table 8.3 Generalized epilepsies

Epilepsy	Old AED	Side effects	New AED	Side effects	Further notes
Juvenile myoclonic epilepsy	VPA PHB	CBZ and PHT aggravate myoclonus	LTG TPM ZNM	VGB and TGB aggravate myoclonus	Lifelong treatment
Idiopathic generalized epilepsy	VPA CBZ PHT PHB		LTG TPM ZNM	VGB and TGB aggravate tonic-clonic activity	
Myoclonic seizures	VPA		TPM LTG KLN		Monotherapy
Absence seizures	VPA ETX LTG	CBZ and PHT aggravate absences	KLN PHB TPM	VGB aggravate absences	Monotherapy
Epilepsy with grand mal on awakening	PHB VPA				Life long treatment
Benign familial neonatal convulsions	PHB PHT VPA				
Benign myoclonic epilepsy of infancy	VPA KLN				Discontinue after 2–3 years seizure freedom; Late treatment can lead to mild mental retardation
West syndrome	ACTH				Good seizure control, cognitive impairment remains
Landau–Kleffner syndrome	VPA KLN or ACTH	CBZ aggravates atonic and absence seizures			Monotherapy or combination
Lennox–Gastaut syndrome	VPA				
Continuous spikes and waves during slow sleep		CBZ aggravates atonic and absence seizures			Monotherapy or combination

ACTH, adrenocorticotrophic hormone; AED, antiepileptic drug; CBZ, Carbamazepine; ETX, Ethosuximide; KLN, Clonazepam; LTG, Lamotrigine; PHB, Phenobarbital; PHT, Phenytoin; TGB, Tiagabine; TPM, Topiramate; VGB, Vigabatrin; VPA, Valproate; ZNM, Zonisamide.

seizures. Benzodiazepines can be used in these patients, however, it is important that tolerance to these drugs may occur. The mechanism of action of the various subtypes of benzodiazepines may differ so that one subtype may be effective when another has failed. Diazepam and lorazepam may induce tonic seizures in some patients. Valproate is less effective in controlling seizures in the symptomatic generalized epilepsies as compared to the idiopathic generalized epilepsies. Other broad spectrum AEDs such as lamotrigine or topiramate can help control some seizure types. Older AEDs such as primidone and phenobarbital may be effective as well, but they are often associated with worsening behaviour such as aggressiveness. Felbamate may also be effective in controlling various seizure types in this syndrome but its risk for liver failure and aplastic anaemia has reduced its role to those patients in whom other treatments have failed. Other methods of treatment include ketogenic diet, VNS, corpus callostomy and ACTH.

Focal epilepsies

Table 8.4 is a brief overview of the standard treatment of the focal epilepsies. Where medical treatment has failed patients should undergo evaluation in the nearest epilepsy monitoring unit for surgery.

Frontal lobe epilepsy

Frontal lobe epilepsy surgery is the second most common surgery performed to treat pharmacoresistant epilepsy. In comparison with other epileptic syndromes it tends to have a non-lesional aetiology making it more difficult to locate the epileptogenic focus; indeed it is prognostically more advantageous when a lesion is identified in neuroimaging studies. Usually invasive studies allow surgery to be performed with a high degree of confidence.

Temporal lobe epilepsy

Patients with mesial temporal lobe epilepsy (**8.1**) will often respond well to treatment with standard AEDs for many years, only to have seizures recur later in life. Surgical treatment provides a good alternative and has been reported to abolish disabling complex partial seizures in approximately 70% of patients. Where pathology is confined to the mesial structures, a resection limited to the mesial structures (selective amygdalohippocampectomy) can be offered in the hope of minimizing additional neurological deficit. However, the potential for this technique in preserving memory has yet to be clinically established. If there is more diffuse pathology a standard temporal lobectomy is often required. In the dominant temporal lobe, the standard resection extends for 3–5 cm behind the temporal pole, in the non-dominant lobe up to 6–7 cm. The most common neurological deficit is a superior quadrantopia, due to damage of the optic radiation that loops through the posterior temporal lobe.

Insular/opercular epilepsy

Insular or opercular epilepsy may masquerade as temporal lobe epilepsy at the time of the initial non-invasive portion of epilepsy surgical evaluation. Clinical semiology, as

Table 8.4 Focal epilepsies

	First-line treatment	Second-line treatment	Further notes
Frontal lobe epilepsy	CBZ		
	PHT		
Temporal lobe epilepsy	VPA		
	GPT	LVT	Monotherapy initially, if
Insular/opercular lobe epilepsy	LTG	PGB	unsuccessful try adjunct
	OXC	TGB	therapy
Posterior epilepsies	PHB	ZNM	
	TPM		
	VGB		

CBZ, Carbamazepine; GPT, Gabapentin; LTG, Lamotrigine; LVT, Levetiracetam; OXC, Oxcarbazepine; PGB, Pregabalin; PHB, Phenobarbital; PHT, Phenytoin; TGB, Tiagabine; TPM, Topiramate; VGB, Vigabatrin; VPA, Valproate; ZNM, Zonisamide.

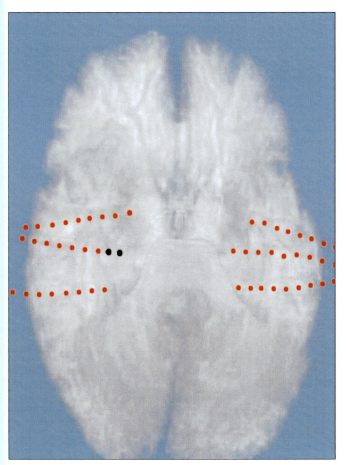

8.1 This shows a three-dimensional reconstruction of the placement of bi-temporal depth electrodes. Sometimes electroencephalography patterns spread so quickly that it is difficult to identify from which temporal lobe the discharges arise from and, therefore, it is necessary to place bilateral depth electrodes to detect the seizure onset accurately.

mentioned in previous chapters, can help guide clinicians to suspect the involvement of these regions. The confirmation of localization to the insula or operculum usually requires the use of an invasive evaluation. As some of these regions are relatively deep, an invasive evaluation with the use of depth electrodes either through SEEG or in combination with subdural electrodes can help identify a focal epileptogenic zone in these deep regions.

Posterior epilepsies

If a structural lesion can be identified accurately (**8.3**) and the epilepsy proves to be AED resistant, these patients may be good surgical candidates. It should be noted that with regards to occipital lobe epilepsy, partially or completely intact visual

fields contralateral to the lesion are considered a significant risk with surgery in this area. Some patients with this form of epilepsy may accept this risk particularly when they are experiencing frequent seizures that are not amenable to medical treatment. Patients with lesions located in the lateral occipital lobe might be spared visual field reductions.

Supplementary sensorimotor area epilepsy

If the epilepsy proves to be refractory to medication and the epileptogenic zone has been identified and lateralized, resection may be considered. Extensive electrophysiological mapping should always be performed before resection to ensure eloquent cortex is not erroneously removed (**8.4**). There are considerable anatomical variations in the precentral sulcus and its relationship with the marginal ramus. Usually a tailored resection following the electrophysiological findings and, if present, neuroimaging findings are used to guide the resection along with eloquent cortex mapping. Some patients display transient and peculiar motor and speech deficits postoperatively, termed as an 'SSMA syndrome'. This syndrome consists of profound weakness of the extremities, accompanied by mutism, particularly with dominant SSMA resections. Many of these symptoms resolve over time.

Overview of the management of status epilepsy

Definitions of status epilepticus vary widely; however, it generally refers to the occurrence of a single unremitting seizure with a duration longer than 30 minutes or frequent clinical seizures without an interictal return to baseline clinical state over 30 minutes. However, the clinical time period for suspected status is 5 minutes as most seizures last only 1–2 minutes. It is imperative that status epilepticus is diagnosed quickly and aggressive treatment started as soon as possible because the longer a patient is seizing the more difficult it is to 'break through' and stop the seizure activity.

The diagnosis of convulsive status epilepticus is usually clear; however, the physician needs a high level of suspicion in cases of altered mental awareness, as this may also be a presentation of subtle status epilepticus. One differential diagnosis to be kept in mind is nonepileptic seizures which

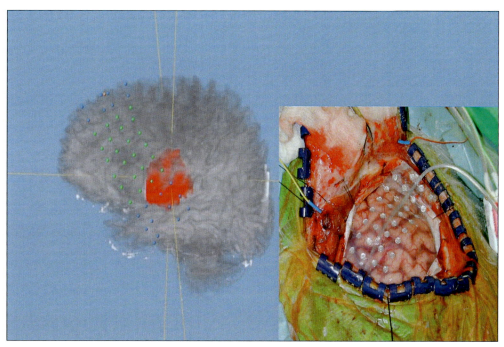

8.2 A three-dimensional reconstruction (left) from magnetic resonance imaging pre-subdural and post-subdural electrode placement with the presence of an insular tumour highlighted in red. Photo (right) taken intraoperatively showing the placement of the subdural electrode grid.

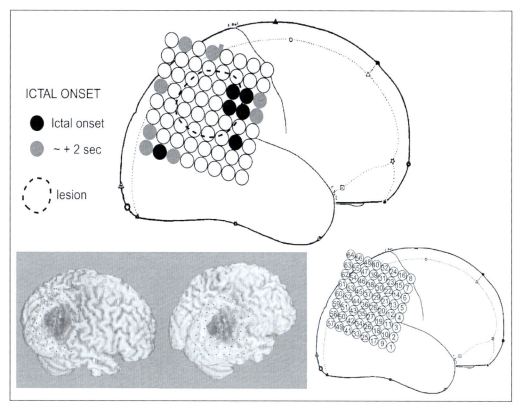

8.3 An invasive evaluation of a lesion seen on neuroimaging, which identifies the ictal onset zone to be in the parietal lobe and corresponding to the lesion.

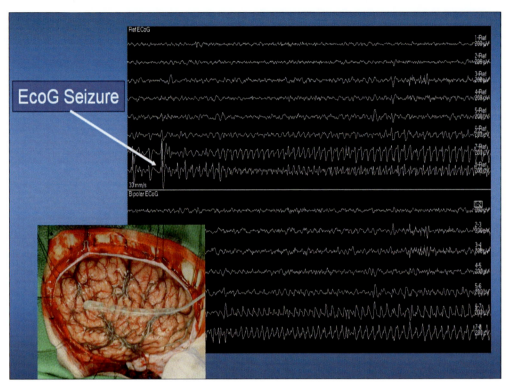

8.4 Placement of one subdural strip intraoperatively and the electrocorticography recording from it, which allows the ictal onset zone to be accurately identified.

can best be confirmed using video-EEG monitoring. The neurological examination in true status epilepticus can yield a variety of findings. If the patient is not in convulsive status with generalized tonic–clonic movements then it is important not to overlook subtle clinical manifestations such as eye twitching, automatic movements or myoclonus. In cases where there is any suspicion of status such as a history of a recent seizure following which the patient fails to return to his/her baseline, an EEG can be very helpful in the diagnosis. An EEG that shows continuous seizure activity is diagnostic of status epilepticus. As with seizures, status epilepticus may be classified under the same headings that were already discussed in Chapter 1 (pages 2–4). It is important to rule out aetiologies other than epilepsy that may lead to severe cerebral dysfunction, such as hypoglycaemia, Korsakow syndrome or herpes encephalitis. Once the airways have been secured and the patient is haemodynamically stable, they should be moved to the intensive care unit.

Malignant status epilepticus refers to status that remains refractory to standard treatments. It occurs in approximately 20% of all status cases and is associated with a poor prognosis.

8.5 depicts a recognized algorithm in the treatment of status epilepticus.

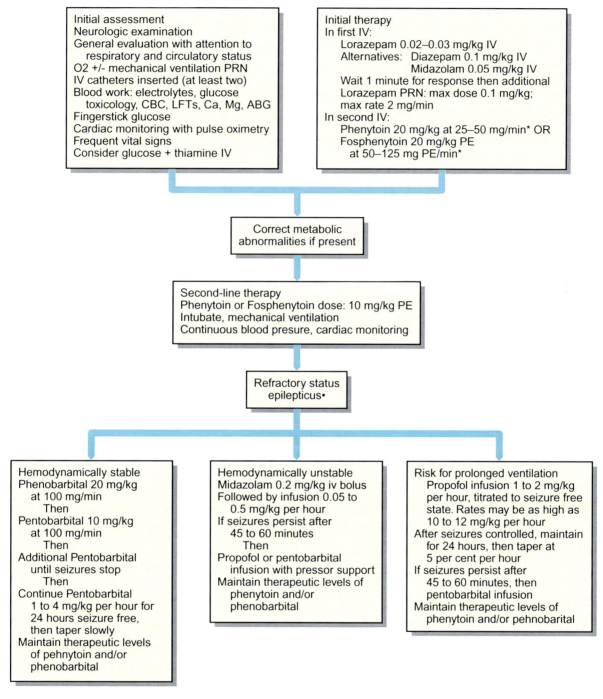

Initial assessment
Neurologic examination
General evaluation with attention to
    respiratory and circulatory status
O2 +/- mechanical ventilation PRN
IV catheters inserted (at least two)
Blood work: electrolytes, glucose
    toxicology, CBC, LFTs, Ca, Mg, ABG
Fingerstick glucose
Cardiac monitoring with pulse oximetry
Frequent vital signs
Consider glucose + thiamine IV

Initial therapy
In first IV:
    Lorazepam 0.02–0.03 mg/kg IV
    Alternatives: Diazepam 0.1 mg/kg IV
                          Midazolam 0.05 mg/kg IV
    Wait 1 minute for response then additional
    Lorazepam PRN: max dose 0.1 mg/kg;
    max rate 2 mg/min
In second IV:
    Phenytoin 20 mg/kg at 25–50 mg/min* OR
    Fosphenytoin 20 mg/kg PE
        at 50–125 mg PE/min*

**Correct metabolic
abnormalities if present**

Second-line therapy
Phenytoin or Fosphenytoin dose: 10 mg/kg PE
Intubate, mechanical ventilation
Continuous blood presure, cardiac monitoring

**Refractory status
epilepticus•**

Hemodynamically stable
Phenobarbital 20 mg/kg
    at 100 mg/min
        Then
Pentobarbital 10 mg/kg
    at 100 mg/min
        Then
Additional Pentobarbital
    until seizures stop
        Then
Continue Pentobarbital
    1 to 4 mg/kg per hour for
    24 hours seizure free,
    then taper slowly
Maintain therapeutic levels
    of pehnytoin and/or
    phenobarbital

Hemodynamically unstable
Midazolam 0.2 mg/kg iv bolus
Followed by infusion 0.05 to
    0.5 mg/kg per hour
If seizures persist after
    45 to 60 minutes
        Then
Propofol or pentobarbital
    infusion with pressor support
Maintain therapeutic levels of
    phenytoin and/or
    phenobarbital

Risk for prolonged ventilation
    Propofol infusion 1 to 2 mg/kg
    per hour, titrated to seizure free
    state. Rates may be as high as
    10 to 12 mg/kg per hour
After seizures controlled, maintain
    for 24 hours, then taper at
    5 per cent per hour
If seizures persist after
    45 to 60 minutes, then
    pentobarbital infusion
Maintain therapeutic levels of
    phenytoin and/or pehnobarital

8.5 A widely used treatment algorithm for patients in status epilepticus, ensuring that patients are haemodynamically stable and receive antiepileptic treatment in a timely manner.

INDEX